Respiratory Disorders and Sleep

Guest Editor

ULYSSES J. MAGALANG, MD

SLEEP MEDICINE CLINICS

www.sleep.theclinics.com

December 2008 • Volume 3 • Number 4

SAUNDERS an imprint of ELSEVIER, Inc.

W.B. SAUNDERS COMPANY
A Division of Elsevier Inc.

1600 John F. Kennedy Boulevard • Suite 1800 • Philadelphia, PA 19103-2899

http://www.sleep.theclinics.com

SLEEP MEDICINE CLINICS Volume 3, Number 4
December 2008, ISSN 1556-407X, ISBN-13: 978-1-4160-6353-7, ISBN-10: 1-4160-6353-6

Editor: Sarah E. Barth

Sleep Medicine Clinics (ISSN 1556-407X) is published quarterly by Elsevier, 360 Park Avenue South, New York, NY 10010. Months of issue are March, June, September and December. Business and Editorial Office: 1600 John F. Kennedy Blvd., Ste. 1800, Philadelphia, PA 19103-2899. Accounting and Circulation Offices: 11830 Westline Industrial Drive, St. Louis, MO 63146. Application to mail at periodicals postage rates is pending at New York, NY and additional mailing offices. Subscription prices are $150.00 per year (US individuals), $76.00 (US students), $339.00 (US institutions), $149.00 (Canadian individuals), $106.00 (Canadian students), $373.00 (Canadian institutions), $185.00 (foreign individuals), $106.00 (foreign students), and $373.00 (foreign institutions). Foreign air speed delivery is included in all Clinics subscription prices. All prices are subject to change without notice. **POSTMASTER:** Send change of address to *Sleep Medicine Clinics*, Elsevier, Periodicals Customer Service, 11830 Westline Industrial Drive, St. Louis, MO 63146. Customer Service (orders, claims, online, change of address): **Elsevier Periodicals Customer Service, 11830 Westline Industrial Drive, St. Louis, MO 63146. Tel: 1-800-654-2452 (U.S. and Canada); 314-453-7041 (outside U.S. and Canada). Fax: 314-453-5170. E-mail: journalscustomerservice-usa@elsevier.com (for print support); journalsonlinesupport-usa@elsevier.com (for online support).**

Reprints. For copies of 100 or more of articles in this publication, please contact the Commercial Reprints Department, Elsevier Inc., 360 Park Avenue South, New York, NY 10010-1710. Tel.: 212-633-3812; Fax: 212-462-1935; E-mail: mailto:reprints@elsevier.com.

Printed in the United States of America.

GOAL STATEMENT

The goal of *Sleep Clinics of North America* is to keep practicing physicians up to date with current clinical practice by providing timely articles reviewing the state of the art in patient care.

ACCREDITATION

The *Sleep Clinics of North America* is planned and implemented in accordance with the Essential Areas and Policies of the Accreditation Council for Continuing Medical Education (ACCME) through the joint sponsorship of the University of Virginia School of Medicine and Elsevier. The University of Virginia School of Medicine is accredited by the ACCME to provide continuing medical education for physicians.

The University of Virginia School of Medicine designates this educational activity for a maximum of 15 *AMA PRA Category 1 Credits*™. Physicians should only claim credit commensurate with the extent of their participation in the activity.

The American Medical Association has determined that physicians not licensed in the US who participate in this CME activity are eligible for 15 *AMA PRA Category 1 Credits*™.

Credit can be earned by reading the text material, taking the CME examination online at http://www.theclinics.com/home/cme, and completing the evaluation. After taking the test, you will be required to review any and all incorrect answers. Following completion of the test and evaluation, your credit will be awarded and you may print your certificate.

FACULTY DISCLOSURE/CONFLICT OF INTEREST

The University of Virginia School of Medicine, as an ACCME accredited provider, endorses and strives to comply with the Accreditation Council for Continuing Medical Education (ACCME) Standards of Commercial Support, Commonwealth of Virginia statutes, University of Virginia policies and procedures, and associated federal and private regulations and guidelines on the need for disclosure and monitoring of proprietary and financial interests that may affect the scientific integrity and balance of content delivered in continuing medical education activities under our auspices.

The University of Virginia School of Medicine requires that all CME activities accredited through this institution be developed independently and be scientifically rigorous, balanced and objective in the presentation/discussion of its content, theories and practices.

All authors/editors participating in an accredited CME activity are expected to disclose to the readers relevant financial relationships with commercial entities occurring within the past 12 months (such as grants or research support, employee, consultant, stock holder, member of speakers bureau, etc.). The University of Virginia School of Medicine will employ appropriate mechanisms to resolve potential conflicts of interest to maintain the standards of fair and balanced education to the reader. Questions about specific strategies can be directed to the Office of Continuing Medical Education, University of Virginia School of Medicine, Charlottesville, Virginia.

The faculty and staff of the University of Virginia Office of Continuing Medical Education have no financial affiliations to disclose.

The authors/editors listed below have identified no professional or financial affiliations for themselves or their spouse/partner:
Murtuza M. Ahmed, MD; Naeem Ali, MD; Raanan Arens, MD; Sarah Barth (Acquisitions Editor); Nitin Y. Bhatt, MD; Himanshu Desai, MD; Michael E. Ezzie, MD; Steven Kadiev, MBBCh; Joseph Kaplan, MD; Meena Khan, MD; Steve Koenig, MD (Test Author); M. Jeffery Mador, MD; Ulysses J. Magalang, MD (Guest Editor); Hiren Muzumdar, MD, MSc; Megan Elise Ruiter, BS; Richard J. Schwab, MD; Daniel R. Smith, MD; Namita Sood, MD; Mark Splaingard, MD; and Karen L. Wood, MD.

The authors/editors listed below have identified the following professional or financial affiliations for themselves or their spouse/partner:
James D. Geyer, MD is an independent contractor and consultant and serves on the Speaker's Bureau and Advisory Board for GSK, serves on the Speaker's Bureau for Cephalon and UCB Pharma, and is an independent contractor and serves on the Speaker's Bureau for Takeda.
Teofilo Lee-Chiong, Jr., MD is an independent contractor for NIH, Restore, Respironics, Schwarz Pharma, and Takeda, and is a consultant for Elsevier.
Kenneth L. Lichstein, PhD owns stock in Sepracor, serves on the Speakers Bureau for Sanofi, is an industry funded research/investigator for Takeda, and is a consultant for Lilly.
John G. Mastronarde, MD is on the Speaker's Bureau for GlaxoSmithKline, Pfizer, and AstraZeneca.
Jonathan P. Parsons, MD, MSc serves on the Speaker's Bureau for GSK and Schering Plough.

Disclosure of Discussion of Non-FDA Approved Uses for Pharmaceutical Products and/or Medical Devices Products.
The University of Virginia School of Medicine, as an ACCME provider, requires that all faculty presenters identify and disclose any off-label uses for pharmaceutical and medical device products. The University of Virginia School of Medicine recommends that each physician fully review all the available data on new products or procedures prior to clinical use.

TO ENROLL

To enroll in the Sleep Clinics of North America Continuing Medical Education program, call customer service at 1-800-654-2452 or visit us online at http://www.theclinics.com/home/cme. The CME program is available to subscribers for an additional fee of $99.95.

Sleep Medicine Clinics

THE CLINICS ARE NOW AVAILABLE ONLINE!

Access your subscription at:
www.theclinics.com

Contributors

CONSULTING EDITOR

TEOFILO LEE-CHIONG, Jr., MD
Head, Division of Sleep Medicine, National Jewish
Health; Associate Professor of Medicine,
University of Colorado Denver School of Medicine,
Denver, Colorado

GUEST EDITOR

ULYSSES J. MAGALANG, MD
Associate Professor of Medicine, Division of
Pulmonary, Allergy, Critical Care, and Sleep
Medicine; Director, Sleep Disorders Program,
The Ohio State University, Columbus, Ohio

AUTHORS

MURTUZA M. AHMED, MD
Instructor in Medicine, Center for Sleep and
Respiratory Neurobiology, University of
Pennsylvania School of Medicine, Translational
Research Laboratories, Philadelphia,
Pennsylvania

NAEEM ALI, MD
Assistant Professor; Medical Intensive Care Unit
Director, Division of Pulmonary, Allergy, Critical
Care and Sleep Medicine, The Ohio State
University, Columbus, Ohio

RAANAN ARENS, MD
Associate Professor of Pediatrics, Division of
Respiratory and Sleep Medicine, The Children's
Hospital at Montefiore, Albert Einstein College of
Medicine, Bronx, New York

NITIN Y. BHATT, MD
Assistant Professor of Medicine, Division of
Pulmonary, Allergy, Critical Care, and Sleep
Medicine, The Ohio State University,
Columbus, Ohio

HIMANSHU DESAI, MD
Fellow, Division of Pulmonary, Critical Care
and Sleep Medicine, Department of Medicine,
State University of New York at Buffalo,
Buffalo, New York

MICHAEL E. EZZIE, MD
Assistant Professor, Division of Pulmonary,
Allergy, Critical Care and Sleep Medicine,
The Ohio State University Medical Center,
Columbus, Ohio

JAMES D. GEYER, MD
Alabama Neurology and Sleep Medicine;
Department of Psychology, The University
of Alabama, Tuscaloosa, Alabama

STEVEN KADIEV, MBBCh
Assistant Professor, Division of Pulmonary,
Allergy, Critical Care and Sleep Medicine,
The Ohio State University, Columbus, Ohio

JOSEPH KAPLAN, MD
Associate Professor of Medicine, Mayo Clinic
College of Medicine; Chair, Division of Pulmonary
Medicine Mayo Clinic Florida; Co-director, Mayo
Sleep Disorders Center, Jacksonville, Florida

MEENA KHAN, MD
Assistant Professor of Medicine, Division
of Pulmonary, Allergy, Critical Care, and
Sleep Medicine, The Ohio State University,
Columbus, Ohio

TEOFILO LEE-CHIONG, Jr., MD
Head, Division of Sleep Medicine, National Jewish Health; Associate Professor of Medicine, University of Colorado Denver School of Medicine, Denver, Colorado

KENNETH L. LICHSTEIN, PhD
Department of Psychology, The University of Alabama, Tuscaloosa, Alabama

M. JEFFERY MADOR, MD
Associate Professor of Medicine, Division of Pulmonary, Critical Care and Sleep Medicine, Department of Medicine, Veterans Affairs Western New York Health Care System and University at Buffalo, Buffalo, New York

JOHN G. MASTRONARDE, MD
Associate Professor; Director, Ohio State University Asthma Center, Division of Pulmonary, Allergy, Critical Care Sleep Medicine, The Ohio State University Medical Center, Columbus, Ohio

HIREN MUZUMDAR, MD, MSc
Assistant Professor of Pediatrics, Division of Respiratory and Sleep Medicine, The Children's Hospital at Montefiore, Albert Einstein College of Medicine, Bronx, New York

JONATHAN P. PARSONS, MD, MSc
Assistant Professor; Associate Director, Ohio State University Asthma Center, Division of Pulmonary, Allergy, Critical Care and Sleep Medicine, The Ohio State University Medical Center, Columbus, Ohio

MEGAN E. RUITER, BS
Department of Psychology, The University of Alabama, Tuscaloosa, Alabama

RICHARD J. SCHWAB, MD
Associate Professor of Medicine, Center for Sleep and Respiratory Neurobiology, University of Pennsylvania School of Medicine, Translational Research Laboratories, Philadelphia, Pennsylvania

DANIEL R. SMITH, MD
Assistant Professor of Medicine, Division of Sleep Medicine, National Jewish Health, Denver, Colorado

NAMITA SOOD, MD
Associate Professor of Medicine; Director, Pulmonary Hypertension Program, Division of Pulmonary, Allergy, Critical Care and Sleep Medicine, The Ohio State University Medical Center, University Hospital, James Cancer Hospital, Davis Heart and Lung Research Institute, Columbus, Ohio

MARK SPLAINGARD, MD
Professor of Clinical Pediatrics, Ohio State University School of Medicine; Director of Sleep Disorder Center, Nationwide Children's Hospital, Columbus, Ohio

KAREN L. WOOD, MD
Assistant Professor of Medicine, Division of Pulmonary, Allergy, Critical Care, and Sleep Medicine, The Ohio State University, Columbus, Ohio

Contents

therapy may alleviate the nocturnal hypoxemia, nocturnal intermittent positive pressure ventilation with or without oxygen seems to improve daytime function and offers a survival advantage in severe disease.

Obesity Hypoventilation Syndrome   525

Meena Khan, Karen L. Wood, and Nitin Y. Bhatt

Obesity hypoventilation syndrome is a combination of obesity, unexplained daytime hypercapnia, and sleep-disordered breathing. It is associated with such symptoms as dyspnea, excessive daytime sleepiness, and impaired cognition. The disorder can result in pulmonary hypertension, severe hypoxemia, cor pulmonale, respiratory failure, and increased mortality. While the etiology is still incompletely understood, the combined effects of obesity, sleep-disordered breathing, and altered leptin levels all likely interact to result in a decreased ventilatory drive. Standard treatment consists of positive airway pressure (continuous positive airway pressure or bi-level positive airway pressure) combined with long-term weight management.

Sleep in Patients with Respiratory Muscle Weakness   541

Himanshu Desai and M. Jeffery Mador

The physiologic effects of sleep on respiratory muscle activity and breathing are described. The evidence of disruption of sleep architecture, SDB and nocturnal oxygenation in patients with respiratory muscle weakness is reviewed. Finally, the more specific findings in various diseases, and the evaluation and management of these conditions, are described.

Pulmonary Arterial Hypertension and Sleep   551

Namita Sood

This article discusses the causes, symptoms, effects, evaluation, and treatment of pulmonary arterial hypertension. It critically reviews the literature concerning its relationship to hypoxia, pulmonary circulation, obstructive sleep apnea, pulmonary hypertension, and overlap syndrome. It points out the need for evaluation of patients with persistent hypoxia or post-treatment symptoms for pulmonary arterial hypertension. Also, it notes that patients with underlying lung disease may not benefit from the standard treatment. It concludes that future studies need to define these conditions and to evaluate patients systematically and using standardized criteria.

Chronic Noninvasive Positive-Pressure Ventilation: Considerations During Sleep   557

Murtuza M. Ahmed and Richard J. Schwab

Noninvasive ventilation (NIV) has become a proven and accepted treatment for respiratory failure from a variety of underlying causes. NIV during sleep can improve gas exchange in both acute and chronic respiratory failure. During sleep, numerous physiologic changes take place that increase the work of breathing and can therefore worsen sleep quality. These include decrements in tidal volume, worsening of gas exchange, and altered lung mechanics. While institution of NIV has been shown to improve nocturnal $Paco_2$ and Pao_2 levels and reduce the work of breathing, less is known regarding its effects on sleep and sleep quality. This article reviews data from case series, uncontrolled studies, randomized clinical trials, and meta-analyses. While there is some controversy, the predominance of data suggests that NIV can significantly improve several measures of sleep quality and duration in patients with chronic respiratory failure from numerous underlying causes. Studies have demonstrated improvements in total sleep time, sleep efficiency, subjective sleep quality, and overall quality of life in patients using NIV. In patients with the obesity hypoventilation syndrome, NIV is a cornerstone of therapy, improving daytime hypersomnolence as well as gas exchange. The data for NIV in patients with chronic obstructive pulmonary disease are conflicting and it is unclear if these patients have overall improvements with NIV use. Implementation of chronic NIV is discussed, along with indications and contraindications to therapy.

The current evidence indicates that acutely ill patients admitted in the intensive care unit (ICU) suffer sleep disturbances that include sleep deprivation (SD), sleep disruption, and, more specifically, decreased or absent slow-wave and rapid eye movement (REM) sleep. Quantifying sleep quality and duration in ICU patients is problematic because subjective and objective sleep measures have inherent weaknesses, and minimal thresholds for sleep have not been established. Sedation and analgesia are often implemented for patient comfort and to provide tolerance to medical interventions and mechanical ventilation. Secondarily, these drugs induce a sleep-like state. However, increased sedation results in disrupted sleep architecture that may impede the normal restorative functions of sleep. Therefore, other interventions should be implemented for critically ill, ICU patients so that restorative sleep can occur.

Following a discussion of the impact of sleep disorders, the clinical management of chronic obstructive pulmonary disorder is discussed, as are asthma and obstructive sleep apnea. Restrictive lung diseases are outlined. The behaviorial management of insomnia appears to improve sleep and the implications are detailed. Finally, the pharmacologic treatment of insomnia for patients who have chronic pulmonary disease is reviewed in detail.

Sleep problems are common in many pediatric respiratory diseases including chronic lung disease of infancy, asthma, cystic fibrosis, sickle cell lung disease, and respiratory insufficiency due to neuromuscular disease and scoliosis. Given the adverse neurocognitive and physiologic effects associated with a deranged night's sleep, the goal of this article is to enhance the physician's ability to anticipate, recognize, and appropriately manage a variety of sleep-related problems including sleep-disordered breathing, gas exchange abnormalities, insomnias, and circadian rhythm disturbances in order to improve children's function and quality of life.

Although respiratory abnormalities and autonomic dysfunction in patients with congenital central alveolar hypoventilation disorders persist throughout life, the prognosis for these children has improved considerably in recent years. This improvement may be attributed to wider recognition of such disorders, specialized centers treating such children, and improved technology to treat and monitor these children throughout life.

Foreword

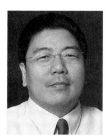

Teofilo Lee-Chiong, Jr., MD
Consulting Editor

Respiration is an automatic behavior that is controlled by metabolic (involuntary) and behavioral non-respiratory (voluntary) processes, such as phonation and deglutition. Both systems operate during wakefulness to maintain adequate ventilation and gas exchange and to achieve optimal levels of acid-base balance (pH), arterial carbon dioxide (Pa_{CO_2}), and arterial oxygen (PaO_2). In contrast, only the metabolic system remains operational during sleep when the wakefulness drive to breathe is inhibited.

Central respiratory neurons, which are responsible for generating respiratory patterns, are active during the inspiratory (active inhalation), post-inspiratory (passive exhalation), or late-expiratory (active exhalation) phases or span different phases of respiration. The ventrolateral reticular formation located in the dorsal brainstem and upper spinal cord includes the pre-Botzinger neurons that are important for the maintenance of the respiratory rhythm; the Botzinger complex late-expiratory and phase-spanning neurons; the ventral respiratory group, which consists of the rostral inspiratory and caudal expiratory neurons; and the upper cervical inspiratory group of neurons. Another respiratory neuron group is located in the dorsal medulla in the ventro-lateral section of solitary tract nucleus. This dorsal respiratory group primarily serves as inspiratory neurons. A pontine respiratory group in the parabrachial region of the dorsolateral pons is not essential for the generation of the basic respiratory rhythm, but lesions in this region can cause an apneustic type of breathing. Finally, the nucleus ambiguous, lying parallel to the ventrolateral respiratory group modulates respiration by its action on the various laryngeal and pharyngeal muscles.

Characteristic patterns of respiration are present during wakefulness, non-rapid eye movement (NREM) sleep, and rapid eye movement (REM) sleep, and each is associated with state-dependent changes in respiratory rate, tidal volume, minute ventilation, and hypoxic and hypercapnic ventilatory responses.

During NREM sleep, respiration is essentially under the sole control of centrally driven metabolic processes. Periodic breathing, with hypopneas and hyperpneas, can occur transiently at sleep onset but may persist into NREM stages 1 and 2 sleep. Breathing eventually becomes regular in amplitude and frequency during slow-wave sleep, as both waking-related respiratory drive and non-respiratory factors affecting respiration are lost. There is a decrease in tidal volume and functional residual capacity during NREM sleep compared to the waking state. Minute ventilation is reduced, resulting in hypoventilation. This, in turn, increases Pa_{CO_2} and decreases PaO_2. NREM sleep also is accompanied by a reduction in inspiratory airflow due primarily to an increase in upper airway resistance, as well as diminished activity of the accessory muscles of respiration, such as the intercostal muscles and the dilator muscles of the nose, pharynx, and larynx.

Further changes in respiration occur during REM sleep, which is characterized by a variable and irregular pattern of respiration, with significant breath-to-breath variability in respiratory rates and tidal volumes. There is generally a further increase in Pa_{CO_2} and decrease in PaO_2.

Sleep Med Clin 3 (2008) xi–xii
doi:10.1016/j.jsmc.2008.08.012

Functional residual capacity is reduced. There is atonia or hypotonia of the upper airway muscles and intercostal muscles due to diminished activity of the motor neurons. On the other hand, activity of the phrenic motor neurons innervating the diaphragm remains intact. Central apneas or periodic breathing may occur, especially during phasic REM sleep.

Finally, ventilatory responses, both hypoxic and hypercapnic, diminish during sleep compared to the waking state. This reduction in ventilatory responses is more pronounced during REM sleep than during NREM sleep. Collectively, these changes in the various respiratory parameters tend to decrease PaO_2 by 2 to 12 mmHg and increase $Paco_2$ by 2 to 8 mmHg during sleep compared to levels during wakefulness.

Changes in respiration also influence the development and clinical presentation of the different pulmonary disorders, including obstructive sleep apnea, chronic obstructive pulmonary disease (COPD), asthma, and restrictive or neuromuscular diseases affecting the respiratory system.

Significant oxygen desaturation can develop during sleep in persons with moderate to severe COPD. Oxygen saturation (SaO_2) normally decreases during NREM sleep compared to levels during wakefulness, and falls further during REM sleep. This is often more pronounced in COPD, where episodes of oxygen desaturation can be more severe, occur more frequently, and be of greater duration. Hypoxemia during sleep is due principally to hypoventilation, but reductions in lung volumes and increasing ventilation–perfusion mismatching may also contribute. Baseline lung function, as well as awake PaO_2 and $Paco_2$ levels, determines severity of arterial oxygen desaturation during sleep.

Nocturnal asthma occurs as a result of an exaggerated decrease in sympathetic activity and enhanced parasympathetic tone during sleep. These, then, give rise to greater bronchoconstriction and increased mucus production. Other mechanisms that may play a pathogenetic role in nocturnal asthma include an endogenous circadian variability in airflow (lowest in the early morning), sleep-related reductions in peak expiratory flow rate, functional residual capacity, minute ventilation and tidal volumes, and alterations in the levels of cortisol, epinephrine, and inflammatory mediators. Increases in total leukocyte count, neutrophils and eosinophils in the bronchoalveolar lavage fluid of individuals with nocturnal asthma have been described.

Persons with OSA commonly have anatomically narrower retropalatal (behind the palate) and retroglossal (behind the tongue) airspaces compared to normal controls. These airspaces narrow further during sleep, which, in susceptible individuals, may result in repetitive episodes of snoring, apnea-hypopneas, oxygen desaturation, and arousals that characterizes obstructive sleep apnea syndrome. Critical closing pressure (P_{crit}) can be defined as the intraluminal pressure at which the upper airway collapses and airflow ceases. Activation of upper airway dilator muscles, which decreases P_{crit}, is diminished by sleep. P_{crit} becomes progressively less negative from nonsnorers to snorers and persons with apneas whose P_{crit} is generally near atmospheric pressure. In addition, sleep blunts the ventilatory response to added inspiratory resistance, which further increases the vulnerability of the upper airways to collapse.

Restrictive lung diseases (interstitial lung disease and kyphoscoliosis) can be associated with significant sleep-related breathing disorders and hypoxemia during sleep. Central and obstructive apnea, as well as hypoventilation, can develop in persons with neuromuscular disorders, such as Duchenne muscular dystrophy, myotonic dystrophy, amyotrophic lateral sclerosis, poliomyelitis, and myasthenia gravis. In both restrictive respiratory diseases and neuromuscular disorders, nocturnal hypoxemia generally predates the emergence of diurnal oxygen desaturation.

It is, thus, made evident in this issue of *Sleep Medicine Clinics* that the sleep state significantly affects the pathophysiology and clinical presentation of many respiratory disorders. Research in the mechanics and cellular biology of the lung must take this into account, as data derived from daytime testing may not necessarily be applicable to the lung during sleep.

Teofilo Lee-Chiong, Jr., MD
Division of Sleep Medicine
National Jewish Health
University of Colorado Denver School of Medicine
1400 Jackson Street
Room J221
Denver, CO 60206, USA

E-mail address:
Lee-ChiongT@NJC.ORG (T. Lee-Chiong)

Preface

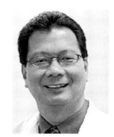

Ulysses J. Magalang, MD
Guest Editor

Respiratory disorders are now the fourth leading cause of death in the United States and affect more than 35 million Americans. Much is known about the symptomatology and management of patients with respiratory disorders during the waking hours, but in recent years, it has become apparent that sleep can have profound effects on the condition of these patients. In this issue of *Sleep Medicine Clinics*, we focus on the effects of sleep on respiratory diseases and the abnormalities that can occur during sleep in those affected by the various types of pulmonary disorders. We have assembled a group of expert clinicians and scientists to offer their perspectives on this important subject.

This issue begins with a general discussion of respiratory physiology during sleep. Sleep in various lung diseases are discussed, including those with obstructive and restrictive abnormalities, as well as respiratory muscle weakness. Separate articles are devoted to obesity hypoventilation syndrome and pulmonary hypertension. Others discuss chronic noninvasive positive airway pressure ventilation, sleep in patients in the intensive care unit, and management of insomnia in patients

with chronic respiratory disorders. Finally, I have invited two experts to discuss sleep in children with respiratory disorders and those with central alveolar hypoventilation syndrome.

I am extremely indebted to the expertise of the experienced clinicians who provide very useful information in this issue. I am particularly grateful to my colleagues at The Ohio State University for their invaluable contribution and advice to the various articles. I am confident that this issue will be a great resource—not only for the busy lung specialist but also for the sleep specialist who will likely encounter these patients in their clinics.

Ulysses J. Magalang, MD
Division of Pulmonary, Allergy, Critical Care,
and Sleep Medicine
Sleep Disorders Program
The Ohio State University
473 West 12th Avenue
Columbus, OH 43210

E-mail address:
magalang.1@osu.edu (U.J. Magalang)

Sleep Med Clin 3 (2008) xiii
doi:10.1016/j.jsmc.2008.09.001

Respiratory Physiology During Sleep

Daniel R. Smith, MD*, Teofilo Lee-Chiong, Jr., MD

KEYWORDS
- Respiratory drive • Control of respiration
- Respiration during sleep • Medications • Asthma
- Chronic obstructive pulmonary disease
- Restrictive lung disease • Neuromuscular disorders

The respiratory system provides continuous homeostasis of Pa_{O_2}, P_{CO_2}, and pH levels during constantly changing physiologic conditions. This elegant system responds promptly to subtle variations in metabolism occurring in both health and disease. During wakefulness, volitional influences can override this automatic control. Modifications occur in the regulation and control of respiration with the onset of sleep. Furthermore, these changes differ significantly with specific sleep stages. Consequences of these alterations of respiratory control can result in the pathogenesis of sleep-related breathing disorders and limit the usual respiratory compensatory changes to specific disease states. This article reviews the normal physiology of respiration in both awake and sleep states, and discusses the effects of common disease processes and medications on the respiratory physiology of sleep.

CONTROL OF RESPIRATION

Ventilatory regulation is conceptually best understood as a three-part system consisting of a central controller, sensors, and effectors. Sensors primarily include central and peripheral chemoreceptors, vagal pulmonary sensors, and chest wall and respiratory muscle afferents. Data from these sensors regarding dynamic oxygen and CO_2 levels, lung volumes, and respiratory muscle activity are continuously transmitted to the central controller. Within the medulla, the central controller generates an automated rhythm of respiration that is constantly modified in response to an integrated input from the various receptors. The controller modulates motor output from the brainstem to

influence the activity of the effectors, namely respiratory motoneurons and muscles. These effectors then alter minute ventilation and gas exchange accordingly.

The medullary ventilatory center consists of neurons in the dorsal respiratory group and the ventral respiratory group.[1] Located in the dorsomedial medulla, ventrolateral to the solitary tract, the dorsal respiratory group was previously believed to be the site of rhythmic inspiratory drive. More recent research in animal models suggests that the respiratory rhythm is generated by a group of cells known as the "pre-Bötzinger complex," a network of cells surrounding the Bötzinger complex in the ventrolateral medulla.[2]

The medullary centers respond to direct influences from the upper airways, intra-arterial chemoreceptors, and lung afferents by the 5th, 9th, and 10th cranial nerves, respectively. The dorsal respiratory group seems to be active primarily during inspiration, with increased frequency of a ramping pattern of firing during continued inspiration. The ventral respiratory group, located within the ventrolateral medulla, contains both inspiratory and expiratory neurons. Ventral respiratory group output increases in response to the need for forced expiration occurring during exercise or with increased airways resistance. Respiratory effector muscles are innervated from the ventral respiratory group by phrenic, intercostal, and abdominal motoneurons.

Poorly understood pontine influences further regulate and coordinate inspiratory and expiratory control. The pneumotaxic center in the rostral pons consists of the nucleus parabrachialis and the Kolliker-Fuse nucleus. This area seems

Division of Sleep Medicine, National Jewish Health, 1400 Jackson Street, Denver, CO 80206, USA
* Corresponding author.
E-mail address: smithdan@njc.org (D.R. Smith).

Sleep Med Clin 3 (2008) 497–503
doi:10.1016/j.jsmc.2008.07.002
1556-407X/08/$ – see front matter © 2008 Elsevier Inc. All rights reserved.

primarily to influence the duration of inspiration and provide tonic input to respiratory pattern generators. Similarly, the apneustic center, located in the lower pons, functions to provide signals that terminate smoothly inspiratory efforts. The pontine input serves to fine tune respiratory patterns and may additionally modulate responses to hypercapnia, hypoxia, and lung inflation.[3] Finally, the automatic central control of respiration may be influenced and temporarily overridden by volitional control from the cerebral cortex for a variety of activities, such as speech, singing, laughing, intentional and psychogenic alterations of respiration, and breath holding.

Afferent input to the central controllers is mediated primarily by central chemoreceptors, peripheral chemoreceptors, intrapulmonary receptors, and chest wall mechanoreceptors. Chemoreceptors provide a direct feedback to central controllers in response to the consequences of altered respiratory efforts. Central chemoreceptors, located primarily within the ventrolateral surface of medulla, respond to changes in brain extracellular fluid [H+] concentration. Other receptors have been recently identified in the brainstem, hypothalamus, and the cerebellum. These receptors are effectively CO_2 receptors because central [H+] concentrations are directly dependent on central P_{CO_2} levels. Central [H+] may differ significantly from arterial [H+] because the blood-brain barrier prevents polar solute diffusion into the cerebrospinal fluid. This isolation results in an indirect central response to most peripheral acid-base disturbances mediated through changes in Pa_{CO_2}. Central responses to changes in P_{CO_2} levels are also slightly delayed for a few minutes by the location of receptors in the brain only, rather than in peripheral vascular tissues.

Peripheral chemoreceptors include the carotid bodies and the aortic bodies. The carotid bodies, located bilaterally at the bifurcation of the internal and external carotid arteries, are the primary peripheral monitors. They are highly vascular structures that monitor the status of blood about to be delivered to the brain and provide afferent input to the medulla through the 9th cranial nerve. The carotid bodies respond mainly to Pa_{O_2}, but also to changes in Pa_{CO_2} and pH. Importantly, they do not respond to lowered oxygen content from anemia or carbon monoxide toxicity. Their mechanisms are integrated, and acute hypoxia induces an increased sensitivity to changes in Pa_{CO_2} and acidosis. Conversely, the response to low Pa_{O_2} is markedly attenuated in the setting of low Pa_{CO_2}.

Respiratory responses to increases in central Pa_{CO_2} levels above 28 mm Hg are linear with increases in respiratory rate, tidal volume, and minute ventilation.[4] Peripheral Pa_{CO_2}-driven responses also vary with differences in levels of Pa_{O_2}. In contrast, the slope of the ventilatory response to Pa_{O_2} varies based on sensitivity and threshold. The response to hypoxia is nonlinear and seems minimal above Pa_{O_2} levels of 60 mm Hg.

Resultant interactions of chemoreceptor inputs regulate normal Pa_{CO_2} levels in humans to between 37 and 43 mm Hg at sea level. In effect, respiratory control is primarily dependent on Pa_{CO_2} with modulation by other factors. Sensitivity of peripheral receptor responses to hypercapnia and hypoxia also increases with a reduction in arterial pH. Whereas acute hypoxia stimulates increased sensitivity to Pa_{CO_2} peripherally, it might depress central respiratory drive.[5]

Additional feedback to the central controller is transmitted from the lung directly from pulmonary stretch receptors and other afferent pathways. Pulmonary stretch receptors are located in proximal airway smooth muscles, and respond to inflation, especially in the setting of hyperinflation. Pulmonary stretch receptors mediate a shortened inspiratory and prolonged expiratory duration. Additional input is also provided by rapidly adapting receptors that sense flow and irritation. J-receptors are located in the juxtacapillary area and seem to mediate dyspnea in the setting of pulmonary vascular congestion. Finally, bronchial c-fibers also affect bronchomotor tone and respond to pulmonary inflammation.

Afferent activity from chest wall and respiratory muscles additionally influences central controller activity. Feedback information regarding muscle stretch, loading, and fatigue may impact both regulatory and somatosensory responses. Upper airway receptors promote airway patency by activation of local muscles including the genioglossus. These receptors may also inhibit thoracic inspiratory muscle activity. Afferent activity enables an appropriate response by central regulation.

The effectors of respiration include the respiratory motoneurons and muscles that are involved in inspiration and expiration. Descending motoneurons include two anatomically separate groups: the corticospinal tracts and the reticulospinal tracts. The phrenic nerve, arising from C3 to C5, innervates the diaphragm as the primary muscle of respiration. Accessory muscles that assist inspiration include the sternocleidomastoid, intercostal, scalene, and parasternal muscles. These muscles serve collectively to stabilize and expand the ribcage. Abdominal muscles are active in expiration and may also assist with inspiration during exercise or in the setting of chronic obstructive pulmonary disease or diaphragm weakness. Finally, upper airway muscles active in inspiration include the genioglossus, palatal muscles, pharyngeal constrictors, and muscles that pull the hyoid anteriorly. Collectively, these muscle groups and motoneurons effect responses generated from central control centers based on input from multiple receptors. This elegant system operates through the complex coordination and interaction of these subcomponents to adapt continuously to changing metabolic needs.

RESPIRATION DURING SLEEP

Regulation of respiration differs significantly between sleep and wakefulness. With sleep onset, there occur important changes in the various processes that regulate respiratory control. Behavioral influences on respiration terminate with cessation of input from the waking state. Positional changes typically associated with sleep also result in significant alterations in respiratory mechanics. Finally, sleep is a dynamic physiologic state with further varying effects on respiration seen in specific sleep stages, particularly in rapid eye movement (REM) compared with non–rapid eye movement (NREM) sleep.

Minute ventilation falls with the onset of sleep in response to decreased metabolism and decreased chemosensitivity to oxygen (O_2) and CO_2.[6,7] Ventilation during NREM sleep demonstrates an inherently more regular respiratory pattern than wakeful breathing, without significant reductions in mean frequencies. The nadir of minute ventilation in NREM sleep occurs during NREM stage 3 sleep (ie, slow wave sleep), primarily as a result of reductions in tidal volume. As a result, end-tidal carbon dioxide ($ETCO_2$) during NREM sleep increases by 1 to 2 torr compared with the waking state.[8] During REM sleep, respiratory patterns and control vary more significantly. REM sleep respiration is typically characterized by an increased frequency and a reduced regularity. Tidal volume is reduced further compared with NREM sleep, resulting in the lowest level of normal minute ventilation. Accordingly, $ETCO_2$ increases of an additional 1 to 2 torr, often associated with a reduction in oxygen saturation, are seen with the onset of REM sleep. Metabolic reductions seen in sleep demonstrate sleep-stage variations with increased rates in REM compared with NREM sleep.

Ventilatory responses to CO_2 and O_2 differ in sleep compared with wakefulness with important distinctions between REM and NREM sleep. The linear increases in ventilatory responses to Pa_{CO_2} persist during NREM sleep, albeit with a reduced slope compared with wakefulness. These changes seem more evident in males than in females, who demonstrate reduced CO_2 responses while awake with less apparent reductions during NREM sleep.[9] In addition, the threshold of the response to CO_2 is shifted upward, with a higher $ETCO_2$ required to drive respiration in sleep. Responses to increases in $ETCO_2$ are further reduced during REM sleep. Respiratory output in sleep, particularly NREM sleep, is significantly reduced in response to hypocapnia. Respiratory responses to hypoxia seem attenuated during NREM sleep, without significant gender-related differences; hypoxia-induced drive is reduced further in REM sleep.

Importantly, both hypoxia and hypercapnea may trigger arousals from sleep, resulting in a return to the more tightly regulated ventilatory control associated with wakefulness. Arousal thresholds for hypercapnia range between 66 and 65 torr and do not vary consistently among the different sleep stages. The threshold for arousal in response to hypoxia is more variable and seems less reliable. Severe oxygen desaturations in some individuals do not uniformly result in arousals.

In addition to the changes in controller responses during sleep, the effectors also demonstrate significant sleep-related functional variation. Of the various effectors of respiration, the upper airway muscles seem to be the most dramatically affected by changes occurring with sleep. These muscles function to maintain patency and prevent collapse of the upper airways during inspiration. These muscles primarily include the genioglossus, tensor palatini, and the sternohyoid, which are active during inspiration during wakefulness and have reduced activity with sleep. The genioglossus responds briskly to increases in Pa_{CO_2} during wakefulness; this response markedly diminishes during sleep. Indeed, the modest increase in Pa_{CO_2} seen with sleep onset does not seem to produce a significant increase in genioglossus activity. In addition, the negative pressure reflex that activates the pharyngeal dilator muscles in the upper airway is markedly reduced during NREM sleep leading to substantial decrements in their activity.[10] Human studies of upper airway responses during REM sleep are limited, with most studies demonstrating that muscle activity is eliminated by generalized REM-sleep associated skeletal muscle atonia; this affect is most prominent during phasic REM sleep. Upper airway responses to hypoxia generally parallel the responses to hypercapnia. Studies consistently demonstrate more striking sleep-related reductions in muscle activity of the upper airway than of the diaphragm or accessory muscles of respiration.

Positional changes during sleep (ie, nonupright position) affect the mechanics of breathing significantly. Upper airway anatomic structures may be more predisposed to collapse, particularly with the concurrent reductions in upper airway muscle tone. Redundant soft tissue–related airway compromise and retroglossal narrowing of the upper airway may be significantly increased in the supine position. Subtle increases in vascular congestion of the airways in response to positional changes may also augment airways resistance. In the supine position, the contribution of chest wall expansion does not exceed the affect of increased abdominal distention, and functional residual capacity is reduced. Intercostal muscle activity is significantly increased during NREM sleep compared with wakefulness and results in proportional increases in chest wall contribution to respiration. With REM sleep–associated atonia, skeletal muscles associated with respiration are significantly impaired and ventilation is accomplished by the diaphragm alone. Chest wall compliance is increased with this decreased intercostal tone, and paradoxical collapse of the chest during inspiration may occur. REM sleep is associated with relative hypoventilation from both reduced respiratory mechanical capacities and decreased sensitivity of the respiratory drive to hypercapnia and hypoxia.

There are significant differences in the responses to increased airways resistance between sleep and wakefulness. During the waking state, increased ventilatory responses to both elastic and airways resistance loading are present; this prompt compensation maintains appropriate ventilation and prevents hypercapnia from developing. Load compensation is significantly reduced during sleep. During NREM sleep, moderate levels of elastic loading (18 cm H_2O/L) results in decreases in minute ventilation and increases in $ETCO_2$.[11] Ventilatory effort is then increased without normalization back to preload levels of ventilation. Lower levels of loading (12 cm H_2O/L) result in significant ventilatory changes over a few breaths with eventual full compensation without arousals.[12] Waking responses to resistance loads include an increase in the duration of respiration, an increase in tidal volume, and a decrease in respiratory rate. Minute ventilation is reduced. Responses to increased resistance during NREM sleep demonstrate a different pattern of reduced tidal volumes, increased respiratory rates, and no significant change in inspiratory time ratio. Reductions in minute ventilation in response to resistance loading are more evident during NREM sleep than in waking states.

MEDICATIONS AND BREATHING DURING SLEEP

There are several drugs that can impair respiration during sleep, including alcohol, anesthetics,

narcotics, and sedative hypnotics. Conversely, some agents, such as almitrine, acetazolamide, some antidepressants, nicotine, progesterone, theophylline, and thyroid hormones, can stimulate breathing during sleep.

Drugs that can Impair Respiration

Alcohol, when ingested while awake, can lead to reduction of both hypoxic and hypercapnic ventilatory responses. Irregular breathing with transient apneas can develop. When ingested close to bedtime, it depresses the upper airway muscle tone and may precipitate or aggravate a pre-existing obstructive sleep apnea; the latter is generally most evident during the first 1 to 3 hours of sleep when alcohol levels are at their highest. Hypercapnia and significant hypoxemia can occur with severe intoxication. The risk of sleep-disordered breathing remains elevated in some abstinent alcoholics following long-term habitual alcohol use, possibly caused by residual upper airway muscle dysfunction or central nervous system damage.[13]

Anesthetics can impair the hypoxic ventilatory response, decrease lung volumes, and decrease upper airway muscle tone, all of which can lead to significant deterioration of respiratory status in patients with an existing obstructive sleep apnea or advanced chronic obstructive lung disease.[14]

Narcotics are potent respiratory depressants and, when ingested at bedtime, can diminish upper airway muscle tone, give rise to hypoxemia, and decrease the hypercapnic ventilatory response.[15]

Sedative hypnotics (eg, benzodiazepines or barbiturates) are mild respiratory depressants. Depression of breathing is more pronounced during coingestion with other central nervous system depressants, such as alcohol, or in individuals with an underlying respiratory impairment (eg, severe chronic obstructive pulmonary disease, neuromuscular weakness, or hypoventilation syndromes). Both agents can decrease upper airway muscle activity and worsen sleep-disordered breathing. They have variable effects on central apneas. Whereas they may increase the frequency and prolong the duration of hypercapnic forms of central apneas (eg, neuromuscular disorders), sedative hypnotics may be beneficial for patients with certain types of nonhypercapnic forms of central apnea, such as those that occur periodically at sleep onset.[16]

Drugs that can Stimulate Respiration

Almitrine is a respiratory stimulant that enhances peripheral chemoreceptor sensitivity. Although it can potentially improve nighttime oxygenation, this effect is generally mild and inconsistent.[17,18]

Acetazolamide administration induces metabolic acidosis from bicarbonate diuresis; this, in turn, can stimulate respiration.[19] Although it is beneficial for the treatment of high altitude–related periodic breathing, its usefulness for patients with obstructive sleep apnea is limited, inconsistent, and unpredictable.

Certain antidepressants, such as protriptyline, a tricyclic antidepressant, and fluoxetine, a selective serotonin reuptake inhibitor, can decrease the frequency and duration of apnea-hypopneas both by increasing upper airway muscle tone and decreasing percentage of REM sleep, during which sleep-disordered breathing tends to be worse as compared with that during NREM sleep.[20] Their clinical use, however, in treating patients with sleep apnea is not established.

Nicotine is a respiratory stimulant. Notwithstanding its effect of enhancing upper airway muscle activity, it has no role in the therapy of obstructive sleep apnea.[21]

Progesterone can increase hypoxic and hypercapnic respiratory responses and minute ventilation; it can improve ventilation in patients with obesity-hypoventilation syndrome and decrease apnea-hypopneas in postmenopausal women.[22,23]

Theophylline can reverse the bronchospasm of nocturnal asthma, increase sleep-related oxygen saturation in patients with chronic obstructive pulmonary disease, and improve Cheyne-Stokes crescendo-decrescendo periodic breathing.[24]

SLEEP PHYSIOLOGY AND RESPIRATORY DISORDERS
Nocturnal Asthma

Patients with nocturnal asthma often present with repetitive arousals and awakenings during the night accompanied by complaints of breathlessness, coughing, and wheezing secondary to bronchocontriction.[25] A variety of factors may contribute to the worsening bronchoreactivity that occurs during sleep, including a relative increase in parasympathetic tone and decrease in nonadrenergic, noncholinergic discharge; comorbid gastroesophageal reflux or obstructive sleep apnea; circadian changes in levels of endogenous hormones (eg, catecholamines, cortisol, or histamine); or reduction of lung volumes and airway size. If severe, nocturnal asthma may give rise to significant hypoxemia.

Chronic Obstructive Pulmonary Disease

Both hypoxemia and hypercapnia can develop during sleep in patients with chronic obstructive pulmonary disease. Respiratory impairment is more severe during REM sleep compared with NREM sleep. Hypoxemia, the extent of which is related to the percentage of REM sleep in relation to total sleep time and daytime levels of Pa_{CO_2}, Pa_{O_2}, and oxygen saturation (Sa_{O_2}), can result from hypoventilation, ventilation-perfusion mismatching, or reduction of lung volume (eg, functional residual capacity). Chronic obstructive pulmonary disease can also occur concurrently with obstructive sleep apnea; referred to as the "overlap syndrome," this is associated with worse hypoxemia and greater pulmonary artery pressures compared with patients with isolated chronic obstructive pulmonary disease.[26,27]

Restrictive Lung Disease

Sleep of patients with interstitial lung disease is often accompanied by frequent arousals; sleep disruption seems to be more pronounced in those with nocturnal oxygen desaturation, the extent of which is influenced by levels of awake Pa_{O_2}, lung compliance, and age of the patient.[28] The increase in respiratory drive present in patients with interstitial lung disease may reduce the prevalence of apneas-hypopneas.

Kyphoscoliosis, by inducing a greater mechanical load of displacing the thoracic cage, can lead to hypercapnia and hypoxemia during sleep.

Obesity is associated with increased work of breathing and greater metabolic demands. Lower functional capacity, less efficient respiratory muscles, and increased mass loading of the thoracic cage (ie, decrease in compliance) can all give rise to hypoxemia, which is generally worse during sleep compared with wakefulness because of the lower functional residual capacity of a supine position, relative hypoventilation, and the development of sleep-related apnea-hypopneas. If severe, obesity can lead to the development of the obesity-hypoventilation syndrome.

Pregnancy, like obesity, can reduce lung volumes (eg, functional residual capacity and residual volume) especially during the third trimester when weight gain and uterine displacement are maximal. Pregnancy may also be associated with an increase in the prevalence of snoring because of structural changes and increased compliance of the upper airways. Apnea-hypopnea frequency and sleep-related hypoxemia tend to be less affected because of the augmented ventilatory drive produced by higher levels of progesterone.

Neuromuscular Disorders

Patients with Duchenne muscular dystrophy can develop hypoventilation and oxygen desaturation during sleep. Myotonic dystrophy can involve the pharyngolaryngeal and diaphragm muscles; obstructive and central apnea-hypopneas, hypoventilation, and oxygen desaturation occurring during sleep has been described. Poliomyelitis is often associated with a defective central control of respiration and can give rise to apneas and hypopneas during sleep. Diaphragm paralysis, especially if bilateral, can lead to increases in $Paco_2$ and reductions in $Pao2$; these derangements in arterial blood gases are generally worse during REM sleep compared with waking and NREM sleep because of the REM sleep-related inhibition of the intercostal and accessory respiratory muscles.[28]

Obstructive Sleep Apnea

Upper airway narrowing and excess weight, if present, can increase the mechanical load on the respiratory system and work of breathing. Oxygen desaturation can result from repetitive episodes of apnea-hypopneas, the latter being more common during REM sleep compared with NREM sleep. Episodes of oxygen desaturation tend to be more frequent and last longer during REM sleep. Hypoxemia and, to a lesser extent, hypercapnia can also arise from the reduction in lung volume related to the supine sleep position (and made worse by comorbid obesity), and augmented respiratory muscle activity generated to compensate for the diminished or absent airflow secondary to upper airway narrowing or collapse (ie Muller maneuver).

REFERENCES

1. Ezure K. Synaptic connections between medullary respiratory neurons and considerations on the genesis of respiratory rhythm. Prog Neurobiol 1990;35: 429–50.
2. Smith JC, Ellenberger HH, Ballanyi K, et al. Pre-Bötzinger complex: a brainstem region that may generate respiratory rhythm in mammals. Science 1991;254:726–9.
3. Mitchell RA, Berger AJ. Neural regulation of respiration. In: Horbein TF, editor. Regulation of breathing (Part I). New York: Marcel Dekker; 1981. p. 541–620.
4. Nattie EE. Central chemosensitivity, sleep, and wakefulness. Respir Physiol 2001;129:257–68.
5. Bisgard GE, Neubauer JA. Peripheral and central effects of hypoxia. In: Demspey JA, Pack AI, editors. Regulation of breathing. 2nd edition. New York: Marcel Dekker; 1995. p. 617–68.
6. Douglas NJ, White DP, Weil JV, et al. Hypoxic ventilatory response decreases during sleep in normal men. Am Rev Respir Dis 1982;125(3):286–9.
7. Douglas NJ, White DP, Weil JV, et al. Hypercapneic ventilatory response in sleeping adults. Am Rev Respir Dis 1982;126(5):758–62.
8. Kreiger J. Respiratory physiology; breathing in normal subjects. In: Kryger M, Roth T, Dement WC, editors. Principles and practice of sleep medicine. Philadelphia: WB Saunders; 2000. p. 229–41.
9. Berthon-Jones M, Sullivan CE. Ventilation and arousal responses to hypercapnia in normal sleeping humans. J Appl Physiol 1984;57:59–67.
10. White DP. The pathogenesis of obstructive sleep apnea. Am J Respir Cell Mol Biol 2006;34:1–6.
11. Wilson PA, Skatrud JB, Dempsey JA. Effects of slow wave sleep on ventilatory compensations to inspiratory loading. Respir Physiol 1984;55:103–20.
12. Badr MS, Skatrud JB, Dempsey JA, et al. Effect of mechanical loading on expiratory and inspiratory muscle activity during NREM sleep. J Appl Physiol 1990;68:1195–202.
13. Sisson JH. Alcohol and airways function in health and disease. Alcohol 2007;41:293–307.
14. Ho AM, Chen S, Karmakar MK. Central apnoea after balanced general anaesthesia that included dexmedetomidine. Br J Anaesth 2005;95:773–5.
15. Wang D, Teichtahl H, Drummer O, et al. Central sleep apnea in stable methadone maintenance treatment patients. Chest 2005;128(3):1348–56.
16. Nickol AH, Leverment J, Richards P, et al. Temazepam at high altitude reduces periodic breathing without impairing next-day performance: a randomized cross-over double-blind study. J Sleep Res 2006;15:445–54.
17. Sans-Torres J, Domingo C, Morón A, et al. Long-term effects of almitrine bismesylate in COPD patients with chronic hypoxaemia. Respir Med 2003;97:599–605.
18. Daskalopoulou E, Patakas D, Tsara V, et al. Comparison of almitrine bismesylate and medroxyprogesterone acetate on oxygenation during wakefulness and sleep in patients with chronic obstructive lung disease. Thorax 1990;45:666–9.
19. Yasuma F, Murohara T, Hayano J. Long-term efficacy of acetazolamide on Cheyne-Stokes respiration in congestive heart failure. Am J Respir Crit Care Med 2006;174:479.
20. Qureshi A, Lee-Chiong TL. Medical treatment of obstructive sleep apnea. Semin Respir Crit Care Med 2005;26(1):96–108.
21. Morgenthaler TI, Kapen S, Lee-Chiong T, et al. Standards of Practice Committee; American Academy of Sleep Medicine. Practice parameters for the medical therapy of obstructive sleep apnea. Sleep 2006;29:1031–5.
22. Javaheri S, Guerra LF. Effects of domperidone and medroxyprogesterone acetate on ventilation in man. Respir Physiol 1990;81:359–70.
23. Saaresranta T, Polo-Kantola P, Irjala K, et al. Respiratory insufficiency in postmenopausal women:

sustained improvement of gas exchange with short-term medroxyprogesterone acetate. Chest 1999; 115:1581–7.

24. Shigemitsu H, Afshar K. Nocturnal asthma. Curr Opin Pulm Med 2007;13:49–55.

25. McNicholas WT. Impact of sleep in COPD. Chest 2000;117:48S–53.

26. Bhullar S, Phillips B. Sleep in COPD patients. COPD 2005;2:355–61.

27. Weitzenblum E, Chaouat A, Kessler R, et al. Overlap syndrome: obstructive sleep apnea in patients with chronic obstructive pulmonary disease. Proc Am Thorac Soc 2008;5(2):237–41.

28. Krachman SL, Criner GJ, Chatila W. Cor pulmonale and sleep-disordered breathing in patients with restrictive lung disease and neuromuscular disorders. Semin Respir Crit Care Med 2003;24: 297–306.

Sleep and Obstructive Lung Diseases

Michael E. Ezzie, MD, Jonathan P. Parsons, MD, MSc,
John G. Mastronarde, MD*

KEYWORDS

- Sleep • Asthma • Chronic obstructive pulmonary disease
- Nocturnal hypoxemia

Obstructive lung diseases are characterized by a limitation of airflow when measured by spirometry. Asthma and chronic obstructive pulmonary disease (COPD) are the two most common forms of obstructive lung diseases. Asthma is defined by reversible airway obstruction caused by inflammation of the lung's airways, often as a response to various triggers. Asthma affects over 14 million adults and 6 million children in the United States.[1] COPD is characterized by airway obstruction that is not fully reversible.[2] It is estimated that 16 million people in the United States have COPD.[3]

Asthma symptoms including cough, wheezing, chest tightness, and dyspnea often worsen at night. Nocturnal asthma is a variable exacerbation of the asthmatic condition occurring at night. Nocturnal asthma is associated with increases in symptoms, worsening of lung function, and increased morbidity. COPD patients often also have increased symptoms at night. It is unclear why asthma and COPD worsen at night, but this may be caused by circadian variations in pulmonary function; inflammation; secretion of hormones; and influences from other concomitant health problems, such as gastroesophageal reflux disease (GERD). Strikingly, both asthmatic patients and COPD patients are more likely to die at night when compared with the general population.[4,5]

It seems that there is also a correlation between sleep quality and the obstructive lung diseases. People with COPD and those with asthma have been shown to have worse sleep quality and more sleep-related problems when compared with people with other chronic health problems. Sleep fragmentation and resultant sleep deprivation can lead to excessive daytime sleepiness and contribute to poor daytime cognitive function leading to social and mental problems. It has also been suggested that there may be a pathologic relationship between obstructive sleep apnea (OSA) and obstructive lung diseases.

This article focuses on the epidemiology, pathogenesis, and clinical implications of sleep disturbances in asthma and COPD, and briefly discusses the diagnostic evaluation and available therapies.

EPIDEMIOLOGY OF ASTHMA AND SLEEP DISORDERS

Approximately 14 to 20 million people in the United States have asthma. In addition, a significant and clinically relevant interaction between sleep and asthma has been demonstrated.[6–8] The interaction is reciprocal, because asthma can affect sleep quality and impact OSA, but sleep-related physiologic changes can also affect the clinical presentation of asthma.

Most asthmatics experience nocturnal symptoms at least once in their lifetimes and many suffer from them routinely. Turner-Warwick[8] surveyed 7729 patients with asthma and found that 74% of respondents experience nocturnal cough and wheeze at least once a week, 64% complained of nocturnal awakenings with asthma symptoms at least three times per week, and 40% awaken nightly. Another study demonstrated asthmatics were twice as likely to complain of difficulty initiating sleep or early morning awakenings, and were

Division of Pulmonary, Allergy, Critical Care and Sleep Medicine, The Ohio State University Medical Center, 201 Davis HLRI, 473 West 12th Avenue, Columbus, OH 43210, USA
* Corresponding author.
E-mail address: john.mastronarde@osumc.edu (J.G. Mastronarde).

Sleep Med Clin 3 (2008) 505–515
doi:10.1016/j.jsmc.2008.07.003
1556-407X/08/$ – see front matter © 2008 Elsevier Inc. All rights reserved.

50% more likely to have symptoms of excessive daytime sleepiness.[7]

In addition to increased symptoms at night and impaired sleep quality, there seems to be a significant relationship between OSA and nocturnal asthma. There is a positive association between OSA; snoring; a history of asthma; and common symptoms of asthma, such as wheezing.[6,8] In addition, there is a positive correlation between GERD and OSA, and the presence of both disorders may exert a synergistic negative effect on nocturnal asthma.[9,10]

PATHOGENESIS OF SLEEP DISORDERS IN ASTHMA

Many physiologic changes that occur normally in sleep may have important consequences related to asthma and may promote nocturnal worsening of asthma (**Box 1**). Several hypotheses have been proposed to explain why asthma symptoms often worsen at night and are discussed next.

Circadian Variations in Lung Function

There is a circadian variation in objective measurements of lung function (**Fig. 1**). Both asthmatics and healthy people experience their lowest peak expiratory flow rates (PEFR) in the early morning hours, usually between 3 AM and 6 AM; however, asthmatics typically have much lower PEFR values indicating more severe bronchospasm.[11] The fluctuations in amplitude from highest to lowest PEFR (PEFR variability) in one study were only 5% to 8% in normal controls compared with 50% or more in asthmatics.[11]

The mechanism responsible for the circadian variability in PEFR and airway resistance remains unknown. Several possible mechanisms have been proposed. One theory suggests that as the body cools normally during sleep, the cooling contributes to nocturnal bronchospasm. Breathing warm, humidified air can reduce the nocturnal

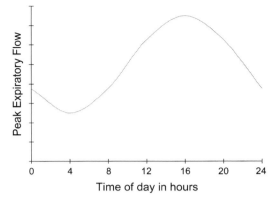

Fig. 1. Diurnal variation in peak expiratory flow rates. Peak flow rates can vary widely in asthmatic patients and often reach their nadir at night during sleep.

worsening of lung function, even if the core body temperature is kept artificially lower, suggesting a direct effect of relatively cold air on the airway.[12] Alternatively, nocturnal symptoms may increase because of prolonged exposure to antigens, such as dust mites that live in pillows and mattresses. A meta-analysis of studies that used physical barriers or chemical strategies to eliminate dust mites concluded, however, that such interventions had no significant effect on morning PEFR or symptom scores. This suggests there may be other antigens in addition to dust mites that must be accounted for and that may play a role in nocturnal symptoms of asthma.[13]

In addition to variations in PEFR, there is a decrease in functional residual capacity (FRC) that occurs during sleep in both normal patients and in patients with asthma. FRC is significantly reduced while supine and sleeping when compared with supine and awake, which suggests that sleep itself is important in the observed reduction in lung volumes.[14] Decreases in FRC may have a significant influence on the increased lower airway resistance that occurs in patients with nocturnal asthma. In addition to decreases in FRC, inspiratory muscle activity is reduced in sleep, which could further contribute to the reduction in lung volumes and increases in lower airway resistance.

Inflammatory Changes at Night

Airway inflammation in nocturnal asthma seems to differ in comparison with nonnocturnal asthma. Bronchoalveolar lavage fluid obtained between 4 PM and 4 AM from asthmatics with nocturnal symptoms has an increase in total leukocyte count, neutrophils, and eosinophils.[15] These and other similar data suggest that the nocturnal

---

Box 1
Physiologic variables that may influence nocturnal asthma

- Airway cooling
- Glucocorticoid receptor changes
- Decreased inspiratory muscle activity
- Decreased peak expiratory flow
- Increased inflammation
- β_2 Receptor down-regulation
- Neuroharmonal changes
- Decreased functional residual capacity
- Increased parasympathetic nervous system activity

worsening of asthma has an associated cellular inflammatory response that is not seen in patients without overnight decrements in lung function.

Inflammation in asthma is typically treated with corticosteroids. Glucocorticoid receptor binding affinity and steroid responsiveness also have circadian variation in subjects with nocturnal asthma.[16] It has been suggested that this may contribute to nocturnal airway inflammation by inhibiting the anti-inflammatory effects of glucocorticoids.

Variation in the Parasympathetic Nervous System

The parasympathetic nervous system has also been implicated in nocturnal asthma. Increased vagal tone during sleep could promote increased bronchoconstriction. There is a diurnal variation in vagal activity that has been demonstrated in asthmatic patients, with higher vagal activity occurring at night. Administration of intravenous atropine to patients in one study with nocturnal asthma produced improvement in the PEFR at 4 AM compared with 4 PM.[17] That study also demonstrated a significant correlation between heart rate and PEFR, which further suggests increased vagal tone at night.

Neurohormonal Changes

In addition to variations in pulmonary function and parasympathetic nervous system tone, there are similar circadian variations in the levels of various neurotransmitters and hormones. Histamine, a potent bronchoconstrictor, has been shown to be significantly higher in asthmatics during sleep when compared with normals.[18] Enhanced nighttime airway inflammation in nocturnal asthma might provide a stimulus for increased endogenous anti-inflammatory activity in the form of increased serum cortisol levels. A blunted adrenal response to corticotrophin, however, which may play a permissive role in the nocturnal worsening of asthma, has been demonstrated.[19] In addition, melatonin, an endogenous sleep-inducing hormone with proinflammatory properties, is higher in asthmatics with nocturnal symptoms as compared with normals.[20] These studies suggest that circadian variation of hormones may play a role in nocturnal worsening of asthma.

Gastroesophageal Reflux

There is a significant association between GERD and asthma.[21–23] Several mechanisms have been proposed to explain the effects of GERD on asthma. GERD is proinflammatory, which can affect the inflammatory environment that is the backdrop of chronic asthma.[21] In addition to promoting inflammation, GERD may exacerbate asthma as a result of direct contact of the esophagus with acid, which has been shown in animal models to be associated with increased respiratory resistance.[24] Furthermore, microaspiration of gastric contents into the airway can lead to vagally mediated bronchospasm.[22] Many patients have worse symptoms of GERD at night because of supine body positioning, which facilitates the entry of stomach contents into the esophagus and airway. This may subsequently exacerbate nocturnal asthma symptoms.

RELATIONSHIP BETWEEN ASTHMA AND OBSTRUCTIVE SLEEP APNEA

There is evidence supporting a positive association between OSA and occasional wheezing, persistent wheezing, snoring, and a history of asthma.[25–27] There are several possible explanations for how asthma may worsen OSA and, conversely, how OSA may complicate asthma.

Sleep Fragmentation

Asthmatics have disrupted sleep architecture as a result of frequent arousals from sleep.[8] Polysomnography in asthmatics has demonstrated increases in spontaneous arousals, decreases in sleep efficiency, and variable effects on sleep stage distribution when compared with healthy controls.[28] Furthermore, evidence also suggests that disrupted sleep architecture may lay the foundation or predispose asthmatics for the subsequent development of OSA. There is a significant association between fragmented sleep and increased airway collapsibility and upper airway resistance indicating that fragmented sleep may lead to early upper airway closure.[29] One can postulate that frequent arousals secondary to nocturnal asthma may unmask or exacerbate coexisting OSA by increasing the magnitude of airway collapse.

Corticosteroid Therapy

Inhaled corticosteroids are the recommended initial controller therapy for patients with persistent asthma symptoms, including nocturnal symptoms.[1] Severe, uncontrolled asthma may require oral corticosteroids. Oral steroid therapy, however, may predispose patients to OSA. An unexpectedly high prevalence of OSA has been demonstrated among patients with unstable asthma receiving long-term chronic or frequent burst of oral corticosteroid therapy.[30] Whether similar effects are seen in chronic, long-term use of inhaled corticosteroids is less well described. It is possible that prolonged and especially continuous oral steroid therapy in asthma may increase upper airway collapsibility possibly by effects on upper airway muscle function and this may play a role in the development of OSA.

Gastroesophageal Reflux Disease

There is a positive correlation between GERD and OSA,[31] and the presence of both disorders may exert a synergistic negative effect on nocturnal asthma. The increased negative inspiratory pressure generated to overcome upper airway obstruction during apneic events may precipitate gastric reflux, which can subsequently exacerbate nocturnal asthma.

Sinus Disease

Sinus and tonsillar inflammation and obstruction, a very common problem in asthmatics, may also play a role in the development of OSA. Nasal congestion from allergies or sinus disease has been suggested to be an independent predictor of snoring in some patients.[32]

Increased Airway Hyperreactivity

Patients with OSA are frequently hypoxic while sleeping. Hypoxia can lead to reflex bronchoconstriction through stimulation of the carotid bodies and subsequent increased vagal tone. In addition, snoring causes repetitive stimulation of the pharynx and glottic inlet, which can also increase parasympathetic tone. Increased vagal tone can lead to nocturnal bronchospasm.[17]

Impaired Arousal Responses

The increased frequency of bronchoconstriction at night can become dangerous because patients with asthma often have poor perception of the symptoms of bronchoconstriction. The response to bronchoconstriction can be further impaired by sleep deprivation, because patients with sleep-disordered breathing have significantly impaired arousal responses to alterations in blood gases.[33,34] Specifically, OSA patients with hypercapnia or hypoxemia have reduced ventilatory responses to hypercapnic and hypoxic stimulation. In patients with both OSA and asthma, the impaired responses to hypoxia and increased prevalence and decreased perception of bronchoconstriction may lead to a vicious cycle of worsening asthma and sleep deprivation and potentially increased morbidity and mortality.

Inflammation

Inflammation is an essential component of asthma and recent data demonstrate that OSA is also characterized by an inflammatory response. Many of the cytokines that are elevated in OSA have also been implicated in the inflammatory pattern demonstrated in asthma.[35] Histologic changes including increased interstitial edema, mucous gland hypertrophy, and infiltration of the uvula lamina propria with T cells in the pharyngeal epithelium in patients with OSA are similar to changes in the bronchi of asthmatics.

RELATIONSHIP BETWEEN NOCTURNAL ASTHMA AND SLEEP QUALITY

Sleep quality is impaired in asthmatics. Specifically, patients with nocturnal asthma have disrupted sleep architecture, more frequent arousals, and report overall worse sleep quality. Positive associations between physician-diagnosed asthma and difficulty initiating sleep, daytime sleepiness, snoring, and self-reported apneas have been reported.[26] Asthmatics are also significantly more likely to report that their sleep is unrefreshing.[25] The presence of impaired sleep quality is clinically significant, because it has been correlated with impaired quality of life and impaired cognitive performance.[36]

Diagnostic Approach

The evaluation of the patient with asthma should include a targeted sleep history in addition to investigation of control of nocturnal symptoms. Frequent wheezing, cough, and bronchodilator use at night are indicators that the patient may need more effective asthma control. In addition, presence and control of syndromes that can worsen nocturnal symptoms of asthma, such as poor sleep hygiene, OSA, snoring, GERD, and allergic rhinitis, should be addressed.

Accumulated data suggest that routine evaluation of the patient with nocturnal asthma should also include a comprehensive sleep history given the poor sleep quality in asthmatics and overlap of OSA and nocturnal asthma. Current guidelines for management of asthma recommend asking about nocturnal asthma symptoms, but do not advise that clinicians take a global sleep history from their asthma patients. If screening questions suggest the possibility of a concomitant sleep disorder, then objective evaluation including such instruments as the Epworth Sleepiness Scale or the Pittsburgh Sleep Quality Index should be considered. If clinical suspicion of a sleep disorder, such as OSA, remains significant, then polysomnography may be required.

Clinical Management

Medical treatment of nocturnal asthma includes control of contributing factors that can worsen asthma including specific environmental control measures, such as plastic covers on pillows and mattresses, adequate ventilation, and optimal humidity in the sleeping environment with minimization of dust. Other factors that are also important in the management of nocturnal asthma include diagnosis and treatment of coexistent medical problems, such as poor sleep hygiene, OSA, gastroesophageal reflux, rhinitis, and sinusitis.

Direct pharmacologic interventions in the treatment of nocturnal asthma include medications that are routinely used in the management of asthma in general. Consideration of optimal dosing levels and timing of administration may be important, however, in the management of nocturnal symptoms.

EPIDEMIOLOGY OF SLEEP DISORDERS IN CHRONIC OBSTRUCTIVE PULMONARY DISEASE

The incidence of COPD has been increasing over several decades and it is projected to be the third leading cause of death in the United States by 2020. Cigarette smoking is the greatest risk factor for the development of COPD and cigarette smoking has also been associated with a high prevalence of sleep-related complaints.[37] Cigarette smoking is associated with a longer sleep latency at onset and a shift toward more stage 1 sleep and less slow wave sleep.[38] Although the exact mechanisms for these changes are not defined, withdrawal from nicotine in cigarettes during sleep may be one of the causes of sleep disturbance in smokers without evidence of COPD.[39]

Patients with COPD have abnormal nocturnal alterations in ventilation and gas exchange.[40] COPD patients with significant daytime hypoxemia (Pa_{O_2} <55 mm Hg) and hypercapnia, often experience a profound drop in nocturnal oxygen saturation, particularly during rapid eye movement (REM) sleep. These oxygen desaturations can exceed 15 minutes and reach nadirs of 60% or lower. Nocturnal desaturations may also occur in non-REM sleep in COPD, but are generally less severe. Nocturnal oxygen desaturations in COPD patients with mild daytime hypoxemia (Pa_{O_2} between 60 and 70 mm Hg) are also common, but the fall in oxygen saturations is mild, with nadir of approximately 88%.[41–44]

Several potential clinical predictors of nocturnal oxygen desaturation in COPD patients have been evaluated. Daytime oxygen saturation, the minimum oxygen saturation with exercise, carbon dioxide retention, forced expiratory volume in 1 second (FEV_1), and elevated body mass index have all been investigated as predictors of nocturnal desaturation.[44–47] Of these, daytime oxygen saturation seems to be the most consistent predictor, with a positive correlation between a resting daytime oxygen saturation less than 93% and nocturnal desaturation.[45,47,48] Both moderate desaturation during exercise[40] and resting Pa_{CO_2} greater than 50 mm Hg have some predictive value, whereas FEV_1 and body mass index fail to predict accurately nocturnal desaturations.

A significant number of patients with COPD experience nocturnal symptoms and these symptoms can fragment their sleep. Klink and colleagues[49] surveyed patients with COPD and found that 39% of patients with nocturnal cough or wheezing reported difficulty initiating or maintaining sleep. If cough and wheezing were both present, 53% reported difficulty initiating or maintaining sleep and 23% reported excessive daytime sleepiness. In addition to increased symptoms at night and impaired sleep quality, there are a number of patients with COPD who also have OSA. This has been labeled the "overlap syndrome," and is discussed later.

PATHOGENESIS OF NOCTURNAL HYPOXEMIA IN CHRONIC OBSTRUCTIVE PULMONARY DISEASE

There is a combination of factors that can contribute to hypoxemia during sleep in people with COPD. Physiologic hypoventilation during sleep is accentuated in COPD and can contribute to nocturnal oxygen desaturation. People who are hypoxemic during wakefulness have resting oxygen levels on the steep portion of the oxyhemoglobin dissociation curve and have a greater fall in oxygen saturation during sleep (**Fig. 2**). In addition to hypoventilation and the role of the oxyhemoglobin dissociation curve, ventilation-perfusion mismatching and a reduced FRC may also play a role in nocturnal hypoxemia in COPD (**Box 2**).

Hypoventilation

During all sleep stages, ventilation is decreased compared with wakefulness in healthy people and people with COPD.[50,51] In healthy individuals during REM sleep, ventilation may be 40% lower than during wakefulness. This is predominantly caused by a reduction in tidal volume. A similar breathing pattern is present during sleep in people with COPD.[52] In people with COPD, however, the physiologic hypoventilation normally present during sleep can result in significant oxygen

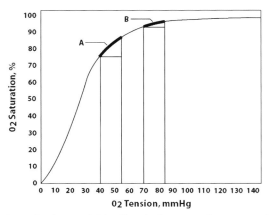

Fig. 2. Oxyhemoglobin dissociation curve in nocturnal hypoxemia. (*A*) In COPD with hypoxemia, there is a greater change in oxygen saturation with a 15 mm Hg drop in Pa_{O_2} because of the steep portion of the curve. (*B*) A small change occurs in oxygen saturation with a drop in Pa_{O_2} of 15 mm Hg in a normal person because this occurs on the flat portion of the curve.

desaturation.[51] In people with severe COPD, oxygen saturation may decrease by 20% during non-REM sleep and may be 40% lower during REM sleep.[53] This is likely a result of the increased physiologic dead space in COPD that leads to an even greater decrease in alveolar ventilation with lower tidal volumes than in normal subjects. This decrease in alveolar ventilation may also lead to a profound decrease in oxygen saturation in COPD patients because of the lower starting point on the oxyhemoglobin dissociation curve.

Hypoventilation during sleep is the result of several factors. There is mild bronchoconstriction during sleep from the normal circadian change in airway caliber, which results in an increase in airway resistance.[11] In non-REM sleep, the basal metabolic rate[54] and ventilatory drive are decreased.[55] These effects may result in a decreased central respiratory drive in non-REM sleep. In REM sleep, the respiratory center has a diminished

response to chemical and mechanical inputs. Additionally, there is hypotonia of skeletal muscles, which includes the accessory muscles of respiration, during REM sleep. People with COPD often are dependent on the accessory muscles of respiration for adequate ventilation, and REM-related muscle paralysis may result in poor ventilation during sleep. The diaphragm is not paralyzed during REM; however, one of the pathologic consequences of COPD is stretching of the diaphragm so that it does not function properly. People with severe COPD may be totally dependent on a poorly functioning diaphragm for nocturnal ventilation.

Changes in Nocturnal Pulmonary Function During Sleep in Chronic Obstructive Pulmonary Disease Patients

The loss of accessory muscle function during REM sleep and the increase in airway resistance during sleep can result in a decrease in FRC.[56] In addition, supine posture is associated with a 10% decrease in FRC in normal subjects.[56] These physiologic changes in pulmonary function, when imposed on people with COPD, may adversely affect the ventilation-perfusion matching and contribute to nocturnal hypercapnia and hypoxemia. In addition, in one study of COPD patients, a decrease in nocturnal ventilation was determined to be the result of a decrease in tidal volume with no change in FRC.[50] Normally, during sleep these changes in lung function and ventilatory drive result in only a small increase in Pa_{CO_2} and usually no hypoxemia.[55] In people with COPD, however, nocturnal changes in ventilation, airway resistance, lung function, and ventilation-perfusion matching may result in significant hypercapnia and hypoxemia.

EFFECTS OF NOCTURNAL DESATURATIONS IN CHRONIC OBSTRUCTIVE PULMONARY DISEASE

There may be marked decreases in oxygen saturation during sleep in COPD that may be more profound than during maximal exercise.[40] The clinical implication of isolated nocturnal desaturations in COPD patients is unclear; however, some physiologic consequences have been documented. Although COPD patients with isolated nocturnal desaturations do not seem to develop pulmonary hypertension,[41] COPD patients with nocturnal desaturations plus mild daytime hypoxemia have demonstrated higher daytime pulmonary artery pressures with possible pulmonary hypertension than in a similar group of patients who did not desaturate at night.[43] The clinical implications, however, of a minor increase in pulmonary artery pressure are unclear.

Box 2
Physiologic changes that may result in nocturnal hypoxemia in COPD

- Hypoventilation
- Oxyhemoglobin dissociation curve
- Increased airway resistance
- Ventilation-perfusion mismatching
- Decreased FRC
- Hypotonia of the skeletal muscles

A combination of factors may contribute to nocturnal hypoxemia in COPD.

In addition to elevated pulmonary artery pressures, there is an increase in premature ventricular contractions during sleep in COPD patients with nocturnal desaturations.[57] The increase in premature ventricular contractions is related to the severity of desaturation because patients with COPD who have nocturnal desaturations to less than 80% show an increase in premature ventricular complex frequency.[58] These premature ventricular contractions tend to decrease in frequency with supplemental oxygen, but the clinical significance of premature ventricular contractions in this case is not established.[57]

It is well documented that among COPD patients with severe daytime hypoxemia, death is more common at night than during the day.[5] It is not clear, however, if there is increased mortality risk associated with nocturnal hypoxemia in COPD patients with mild daytime hypoxemia because studies have been conflicted.[59,60]

RELATIONSHIP BETWEEN CHRONIC OBSTRUCTIVE PULMONARY DISEASE AND OBSTRUCTIVE SLEEP APNEA

COPD and OSA are both common diseases and both conditions could be expected to occur in the same individual by chance. When this occurs, it has been termed "the overlap syndrome." There have been several studies that have examined the association between COPD and OSA.[61–64] A study of 265 patients referred to a sleep laboratory for various reasons found 11% to have obstructive lung disease by spirometry.[63] At the time, this was a higher prevalence than expected in the general population and suggested there may be a pathologic link between the two diseases. In the Sleep Heart Health study, however, participants with obstructive airways disease as defined purely by spirometry (FEV_1/forced vital capacity <70%) had a prevalence of sleep apnea (Respiratory Disturbance Index >10) of 22.3% versus 28.9% in participants with normal spirometry.[65] Moreover, there was minimal alteration in sleep quality in those with obstruction.[65] These authors proposed that when obstructive airways disease and OSA occur in the same individual it is by chance and there is no pathophysiologic link between the two disorders. This study was limited by a low percentage of subjects with severe obstructive airways disease and by reliance solely on a single spirometry for the diagnosis of chronic obstructive lung disease. Although a pathologic link between the two diseases may or may not exist, it is clear that when they coexist patients may display more profound nocturnal desaturations and worsened sleep quality. In addition, patients with the overlap syndrome may be more prone to the development of pulmonary hypertension, especially if they have daytime hypoxemia.[66] In general, people with COPD do not develop pulmonary hypertension unless they have severe obstruction with significant hypoxemia. People with the overlap syndrome can develop pulmonary hypertension, however, with only mild to moderate obstruction. This may result from the combined effects of both diseases contributing to hypoxemia and effects on pulmonary hemodynamics.

CHRONIC OBSTRUCTIVE PULMONARY DISEASE AND SLEEP QUALITY

There have been several studies demonstrating that people with COPD have worse sleep quality compared with healthy individuals.[67–69] There is a higher prevalence of insomnia, use of hypnotic medications, and an increase in daytime sleepiness in people with COPD than the general population.[69,70] The exact mechanisms of these sleep disturbances in COPD are not clear, but there have been several studies evaluating sleep architecture in COPD patients.

Studies using polysomnography have documented sleep fragmentation with frequent arousals, less total sleep time, and less slow wave and REM sleep in people with COPD compared with healthy controls.[71,72] In the Sleep Heart Health Study, however, people with mild obstructive airways disease without OSA were not sleepier by the Epworth Sleepiness Scale than those without obstructive airways disease. Furthermore, people with obstructive airways disease had no significant differences in sleep architecture compared with those without obstructive airways disease and OSA.[65] Participants with the overlap syndrome had higher Epworth sleepiness scores, lower total sleep time, lower sleep efficiency, and a higher arousal index compared with those with obstructive airways disease alone, however, but there was only a small difference between those with OSA alone and those with the overlap syndrome.[65] It seems that in patients with mild obstructive airways disease there is little effect on sleep quality. As obstructive lung disease becomes more severe, however, there are increased sleep complaints. In addition, when OSA is superimposed on obstructive lung disease there are more sleep complaints and possibly more deleterious physiologic effects.

Diagnostic Approach

Patients with COPD should be questioned about global sleep issues with particular emphasis on symptoms of sleep apnea including daytime hypersomnolence, morning headaches, snoring, and witnessed apneas. If symptoms are found, these patients should undergo polysomnography testing. In addition, the Global Initiative for Obstructive Lung Disease (GOLD) guidelines recommend evaluation by polysomnography when hypoxemia or right heart failure develops in COPD in the presence of relatively mild airflow limitation.[73] The overlap syndrome may contribute to pulmonary artery pressure elevations in these patients. If there is concern for nocturnal desaturations alone based on oxygen saturations less than 93% during the day, this may be evaluated by a simple nocturnal oximetry. Nocturnal oximetry may also be used to evaluate the effectiveness of oxygen therapy in improving oxygen saturations.

Clinical Management

The best practices for management of COPD may also improve nocturnal hypoxemia. Anticholinergics have been shown to improve nocturnal oxygenation and sleep quality in COPD.[74,75] Theophylline, however, may improve gas exchange but studies conflict regarding the effect on the quality of sleep in COPD.[76–78] Other medications that have been studied in COPD for nocturnal hypoxemia including medroxyprogesterone acetate, acetazolamide, almitrine, and protriptyline have all been limited by side effects and lack strong supportive data. COPD patients with either severe COPD or hypercapnia should avoid hypnotics and alcohol, which may decrease respiratory drive with resultant hypercapneic respiratory failure. There is evidence that zolpidem does not decrease respiratory drive or minute ventilation in patients with COPD and might be a useful sleep aid.[79,80]

The clinical question of what level of nocturnal hypoxemia in COPD warrants treatment is controversial and lacks firm evidence-based recommendation. The Nocturnal Oxygen Therapy Trial and the Medical Research Council Working Party both showed improved survival with long-term oxygen therapy that included use during sleep; however, they did not target people with isolated nocturnal desaturations.[61,81] Currently, the GOLD guidelines recommend that nocturnal oxygen therapy should be provided to patients whose oxygen saturations fall below 88% or who have a Pao_2 less than 55 mm Hg during wakefulness. This is based on B level evidence (limited body of data from randomized controlled trials).[73] The primary goal of oxygen administration is to increase the baseline Pao_2 to 60 mm Hg or an Spo_2 of 90% during the day.[73] Caution is needed when instituting oxygen therapy in those with daytime hypercapnia.

Daytime arterial blood gas determinations should be considered soon after instituting oxygen to evaluate for worsening hypercapnia. There are no current recommendations from the GOLD committee on nocturnal oxygen management because there are ongoing trials in this area. Noninvasive positive pressure ventilation in combination with oxygen therapy may be of benefit to a subset of patients with daytime hypercapnia, but more studies are needed before this can be recommended for routine clinical practice.[73] Lung volume reduction surgery also results in improved sleep quality and nocturnal oxygenation in severe COPD and further long-term outcomes are awaited from current trials.[82]

SUMMARY

Obstructive lung diseases and sleep disorders are both common conditions with a complex intertwined relationship. The factors that contribute to worsened symptoms and oxygenation at night in asthma and COPD are not completely understood. In addition, asthma and COPD and OSA result in disrupted sleep architecture and decreased sleep quality. It is important as a clinician to recognize that management of the patient with obstructive lung disease should include a comprehensive sleep history including sleep hygiene, symptoms of GERD, sinus disease, and OSA. Recognition of sleep-related disturbances in patients with obstructive lung disease assists clinicians in the management of their patients and allows for improved respiratory and sleep-related quality of life.

REFERENCES

1. National Heart Lung and Blood Institute. Expert Panel Report 3 (EPR3): guidelines for the diagnosis and management of asthma. Available at: http://www.nhlbi.nih.gov/guidelines/asthma/asthgdln.htm. Accessed October 1, 2008.
2. Pauwels RA, Buist AS, Calverley PM, et al. Global strategy for the diagnosis, management, and prevention of chronic obstructive pulmonary disease. NHLBI/WHO Global Initiative for Chronic Obstructive Lung Disease (GOLD) Workshop summary. Am J Respir Crit Care Med 2001;163:1256–76.
3. Adams PF, Hendershot GE, Marano MA. Current estimates from the National Health Interview Survey, 1996. Vital Health Stat 10 1999;10:1–203.
4. Hetzel MR, Clark TJ, Branthwaite MA. Asthma: analysis of sudden deaths and ventilatory arrests in hospital. Br Med J 1977;1:808–11.
5. McNicholas WT, Fitzgerald MX. Nocturnal deaths among patients with chronic bronchitis and emphysema. Br Med J (Clin Res Ed) 1984;289:878.

6. Ekici A, Ekici M, Kurtipek E, et al. Association of asthma-related symptoms with snoring and apnea and effect on health-related quality of life. Chest 2005;128:3358–63.

7. Lewis DA. Sleep in patients with asthma and chronic obstructive pulmonary disease. Curr Opin Pulm Med 2001;7:105–12.

8. Turner-Warwick M. Epidemiology of nocturnal asthma. Am J Med 1988;85:6–8.

9. Harding SM. Gastroesophageal reflux: a potential asthma trigger. Immunol Allergy Clin North Am 2005;25:131–48.

10. Kasasbeh A, Kasasbeh E, Krishnaswamy G. Potential mechanisms connecting asthma, esophageal reflux, and obesity/sleep apnea complex: a hypothetical review. Sleep Med Rev 2007;11:47–58.

11. Hetzel MR, Clark TJ. Comparison of normal and asthmatic circadian rhythms in peak expiratory flow rate. Thorax 1980;35:732–8.

12. Chen WY, Chai H. Airway cooling and nocturnal asthma. Chest 1982;81:675–80.

13. Hammarquist C, Burr ML, Gotzsche PC. House dust mite control measures for asthma. Cochrane Database Syst Rev 2000;CD001187.

14. Ballard RD, Irvin CG, Martin RJ, et al. Influence of sleep on lung volume in asthmatic patients and normal subjects. J Appl Physiol 1990;68:2034–41.

15. Kraft M, Djukanovic R, Wilson S, et al. Alveolar tissue inflammation in asthma. Am J Respir Crit Care Med 1996;154:1505–10.

16. Kraft M, Vianna E, Martin RJ, et al. Nocturnal asthma is associated with reduced glucocorticoid receptor binding affinity and decreased steroid responsiveness at night. J Allergy Clin Immunol 1999;103:66–71.

17. Morrison JF, Pearson SB. The effect of the circadian rhythm of vagal activity on bronchomotor tone in asthma. Br J Clin Pharmacol 1989;28:545–9.

18. Szefler SJ, Ando R, Cicutto LC, et al. Plasma histamine, epinephrine, cortisol, and leukocyte beta-adrenergic receptors in nocturnal asthma. Clin Pharmacol Ther 1991;49:59–68.

19. Sutherland ER, Ellison MC, Kraft M, et al. Altered pituitary-adrenal interaction in nocturnal asthma. J Allergy Clin Immunol 2003;112:52–7.

20. Sutherland ER, Martin RJ. Airway inflammation in chronic obstructive pulmonary disease: comparisons with asthma. J Allergy Clin Immunol 2003;112:819–27.

21. Hamamoto J, Kohrogi H, Kawano O, et al. Esophageal stimulation by hydrochloric acid causes neurogenic inflammation in the airways in guinea pigs. J Appl Physiol 1997;82:738–45.

22. Jack CI, Calverley PM, Donnelly RJ, et al. Simultaneous tracheal and oesophageal pH measurements in asthmatic patients with gastro-oesophageal reflux. Thorax 1995;50:201–4.

23. Mansfield LE, Stein MR. Gastroesophageal reflux and asthma: a possible reflex mechanism. Ann Allergy 1978;41:224–6.

24. Mansfield LE, Hameister HH, Spaulding HS, et al. The role of the vague nerve in airway narrowing caused by intraesophageal hydrochloric acid provocation and esophageal distention. Ann Allergy 1981;47:431–4.

25. Fitzpatrick MF, Martin K, Fossey E, et al. Snoring, asthma and sleep disturbance in Britain: a community-based survey. Eur Respir J 1993;6:531–5.

26. Janson C, De Backer W, Gislason T, et al. Increased prevalence of sleep disturbances and daytime sleepiness in subjects with bronchial asthma: a population study of young adults in three European countries. Eur Respir J 1996;9:2132–8.

27. Janson C, Gislason T, De Backer W, et al. Prevalence of sleep disturbances among young adults in three European countries. Sleep 1995;18:589–97.

28. Montplaisir J, Walsh J, Malo JL. Nocturnal asthma: features of attacks, sleep and breathing patterns. Am Rev Respir Dis 1982;125:18–22.

29. Series F, Roy N, Marc I. Effects of sleep deprivation and sleep fragmentation on upper airway collapsibility in normal subjects. Am J Respir Crit Care Med 1994;150:481–5.

30. Yigla M, Tov N, Solomonov A, et al. Difficult-to-control asthma and obstructive sleep apnea. J Asthma 2003;40:865–71.

31. Orr WC, Heading R, Johnson LF, et al. Review article: sleep and its relationship to gastro-oesophageal reflux. Aliment Pharmacol Ther 2004;20(Suppl 9):39–46.

32. Larsson LG, Lindberg A, Franklin KA, et al. Symptoms related to obstructive sleep apnoea are common in subjects with asthma, chronic bronchitis and rhinitis in a general population. Respir Med 2001;95:423–9.

33. Ballard RD, Saathoff MC, Patel DK, et al. Effect of sleep on nocturnal bronchoconstriction and ventilatory patterns in asthmatics. J Appl Physiol 1989;67:243–9.

34. Ballard RD, Tan WC, Kelly PL, et al. Effect of sleep and sleep deprivation on ventilatory response to bronchoconstriction. J Appl Physiol 1990;69:490–7.

35. Busse WW, Lemanske RF Jr. Asthma. N Engl J Med 2001;344:350–62.

36. Aldrich M. Impact, presentation and diagnosis. In: Kryger MH, Roth T, Dement WC, editors. Principles and practice of sleep medicine. Philadelphia: WB Sanders; 2000. p. 521–80.

37. Phillips BA, Danner FJ. Cigarette smoking and sleep disturbance. Arch Intern Med 1995;155:734–7.

38. Zhang L, Samet J, Caffo B, et al. Cigarette smoking and nocturnal sleep architecture. Am J Epidemiol 2006;164:529–37.

39. Zhang L, Samet J, Caffo B, et al. Power spectral analysis of EEG activity during sleep in cigarette smokers. Chest 2008;133:427–32.

40. Mulloy E, McNicholas WT. Ventilation and gas exchange during sleep and exercise in severe COPD. Chest 1996;109:387–94.

41. Chaouat A, Weitzenblum E, Kessler R, et al. Sleep-related O2 desaturation and daytime pulmonary haemodynamics in COPD patients with mild hypoxaemia. Eur Respir J 1997;10:1730–5.

42. Fletcher EC, Miller J, Divine GW, et al. Nocturnal oxyhemoglobin desaturation in COPD patients with arterial oxygen tensions above 60 mm Hg. Chest 1987;92:604–8.

43. Levi-Valensi P, Weitzenblum E, Rida Z, et al. Sleep-related oxygen desaturation and daytime pulmonary haemodynamics in COPD patients. Eur Respir J 1992;5:301–7.

44. Vos PJ, Folgering HT, van Herwaarden CL. Predictors for nocturnal hypoxaemia (mean SaO2 < 90%) in normoxic and mildly hypoxic patients with COPD. Eur Respir J 1995;8:74–7.

45. Thomas VD, Vinod Kumar S, Gitanjali B. Predictors of nocturnal oxygen desaturation in chronic obstructive pulmonary disease in a South Indian population. J Postgrad Med 2002;48:101–4.

46. Toraldo DM, Nicolardi G, De Nuccio F, et al. Pattern of variables describing desaturator COPD patients, as revealed by cluster analysis. Chest 2005;128:3828–37.

47. Little SA, Elkholy MM, Chalmers GW, et al. Predictors of nocturnal oxygen desaturation in patients with COPD. Respir Med 1999;93:202–7.

48. Weitzenblum E, Chaouat A. Sleep and chronic obstructive pulmonary disease. Sleep Med Rev 2004;8:281–94.

49. Klink ME, Dodge R, Quan SF. The relation of sleep complaints to respiratory symptoms in a general population. Chest 1994;105:151–4.

50. Ballard RD, Clover CW, Suh BY. Influence of sleep on respiratory function in emphysema. Am J Respir Crit Care Med 1995;151:945–51.

51. Hudgel DW, Martin RJ, Capehart M, et al. Contribution of hypoventilation to sleep oxygen desaturation in chronic obstructive pulmonary disease. J Appl Physiol 1983;55:669–77.

52. Catterall JR, Douglas NJ, Calverley PM, et al. Transient hypoxemia during sleep in chronic obstructive pulmonary disease is not a sleep apnea syndrome. Am Rev Respir Dis 1983;128:24–9.

53. Becker HF, Piper AJ, Flynn WE, et al. Breathing during sleep in patients with nocturnal desaturation. Am J Respir Crit Care Med 1999;159:112–8.

54. White DP, Weil JV, Zwillich CW. Metabolic rate and breathing during sleep. J Appl Physiol 1985;59:384–91.

55. Meurice JC, Marc I, Series F. Influence of sleep on ventilatory and upper airway response to CO2 in normal subjects and patients with COPD. Am J Respir Crit Care Med 1995;152:1620–6.

56. Hudgel DW, Devadatta P. Decrease in functional residual capacity during sleep in normal humans. J Appl Physiol 1984;57:1319–22.

57. Tirlapur VG, Mir MA. Nocturnal hypoxemia and associated electrocardiographic changes in patients with chronic obstructive airways disease. N Engl J Med 1982;306:125–30.

58. Shepard JW Jr, Garrison MW, Grither DA, et al. Relationship of ventricular ectopy to nocturnal oxygen desaturation in patients with chronic obstructive pulmonary disease. Am J Med 1985;78:28–34.

59. Chaouat A, Weitzenblum E, Kessler R, et al. A randomized trial of nocturnal oxygen therapy in chronic obstructive pulmonary disease patients. Eur Respir J 1999;14:1002–8.

60. Fletcher EC, Donner CF, Midgren B, et al. Survival in COPD patients with a daytime PaO2 greater than 60 mm Hg with and without nocturnal oxyhemoglobin desaturation. Chest 1992;101:649–55.

61. Nocturnal Oxygen Therapy Trial Group. Continuous or nocturnal oxygen therapy in hypoxemic chronic obstructive lung disease: a clinical trial. Ann Intern Med 1980;93:391–8.

62. Brander PE, Kuitunen T, Salmi T, et al. Nocturnal oxygen saturation in advanced chronic obstructive pulmonary disease after a moderate dose of ethanol. Eur Respir J 1992;5:308–12.

63. Chaouat A, Weitzenblum E, Krieger J, et al. Association of chronic obstructive pulmonary disease and sleep apnea syndrome. Am J Respir Crit Care Med 1995;151:82–6.

64. O'Donoghue FJ, Catcheside PG, Ellis EE, et al. Sleep hypoventilation in hypercapnic chronic obstructive pulmonary disease: prevalence and associated factors. Eur Respir J 2003;21:977–84.

65. Sanders MH, Newman AB, Haggerty CL, et al. Sleep and sleep-disordered breathing in adults with predominantly mild obstructive airway disease. Am J Respir Crit Care Med 2003;167:7–14.

66. Weitzenblum E, Krieger J, Apprill M, et al. Daytime pulmonary hypertension in patients with obstructive sleep apnea syndrome. Am Rev Respir Dis 1988;138:345–9.

67. Brezinova V, Catterall JR, Douglas NJ, et al. Night sleep of patients with chronic ventilatory failure and age matched controls: number and duration of the EEG episodes of intervening wakefulness and drowsiness. Sleep 1982;5:123–30.

68. Calverley PM, Brezinova V, Douglas NJ, et al. The effect of oxygenation on sleep quality in chronic bronchitis and emphysema. Am Rev Respir Dis 1982;126:206–10.

69. Fleetham J, West P, Mezon B, et al. Sleep, arousals, and oxygen desaturation in chronic obstructive pulmonary disease: the effect of oxygen therapy. Am Rev Respir Dis 1982;126:429–33.

70. Klink M, Quan SF. Prevalence of reported sleep disturbances in a general adult population and their relationship to obstructive airways diseases. Chest 1987;91:540–6.

71. Cormick W, Olson LG, Hensley MJ, et al. Nocturnal hypoxaemia and quality of sleep in patients with chronic obstructive lung disease. Thorax 1986;41:846–54.

72. Sandek K, Andersson T, Bratel T, et al. Sleep quality, carbon dioxide responsiveness and hypoxaemic patterns in nocturnal hypoxaemia due to chronic obstructive pulmonary disease (COPD) without daytime hypoxaemia. Respir Med 1999;93:79–87.

73. Rabe KF, Hurd S, Anzueto A, et al. Global strategy for the diagnosis, management, and prevention of chronic obstructive pulmonary disease: GOLD executive summary. Am J Respir Crit Care Med 2007;176:532–55.

74. Martin RJ, Bartelson BL, Smith P, et al. Effect of ipratropium bromide treatment on oxygen saturation and sleep quality in COPD. Chest 1999;115:1338–45.

75. McNicholas WT, Calverley PM, Lee A, et al. Long-acting inhaled anticholinergic therapy improves sleeping oxygen saturation in COPD. Eur Respir J 2004;23:825–31.

76. Mulloy E, McNicholas WT. Theophylline improves gas exchange during rest, exercise, and sleep in severe chronic obstructive pulmonary disease. Am Rev Respir Dis 1993;148:1030–6.

77. Man GC, Champman KR, Ali SH, et al. Sleep quality and nocturnal respiratory function with once-daily theophylline (Uniphyl) and inhaled salbutamol in patients with COPD. Chest 1996;110:648–53.

78. Martin RJ, Pak J. Overnight theophylline concentrations and effects on sleep and lung function in chronic obstructive pulmonary disease. Am Rev Respir Dis 1992;145:540–4.

79. Murciano D, Armengaud MH, Cramer PH, et al. Acute effects of zolpidem, triazolam and flunitrazepam on arterial blood gases and control of breathing in severe COPD. Eur Respir J 1993;6:625–9.

80. Steens RD, Pouliot Z, Millar TW, et al. Effects of zolpidem and triazolam on sleep and respiration in mild to moderate chronic obstructive pulmonary disease. Sleep 1993;16:318–26.

81. Medical Research Council Working Party. Long term domiciliary oxygen therapy in chronic hypoxic cor pulmonale complicating chronic bronchitis and emphysema: report of the Medical Research Council Working Party. Lancet 1981;1:681–6.

82. Krachman SL, Chatila W, Martin UJ, et al. Effects of lung volume reduction surgery on sleep quality and nocturnal gas exchange in patients with severe emphysema. Chest 2005;128:3221–8.

Sleep and Breathing in Restrictive Thoracic Cage and Lung Disease

Joseph Kaplan, MD

KEYWORDS

- Sleep • Kyphoscoliosis • Interstitial lung disease
- Chronic respiratory failure • Noninvasive ventilation

Restriction in pulmonary function is characterized by a reduction in absolute lung volumes (total lung capacity, functional residual capacity, vital capacity, and expiratory reserve volume) with preservation or even augmentation of flow rates (reflected in the ratio of the forced expiratory volume in 1 second divided by the forced vital capacity, the peak flow, and the maximum midexpiratory flow). Typically, the diffusing capacity is reduced commensurate with the reductions in lung volumes. Intrapulmonary restriction involves disease of the pulmonary parenchyma; usually interstitial lung disease (ILD) and extrapulmonary restriction involves abnormalities of the pleura or chest wall. Obesity represents a subtype of restrictive disease and is discussed elsewhere in this issue.

INTRAPULMONARY RESTRICTION: INTERSTITIAL LUNG DISEASE

Restriction in ILD is characterized by abnormalities in lung mechanics and gas exchange. Common pathologic changes in the pulmonary parenchyma include alveolar thickening caused by fibrosis, cellular exudates, and edema. Alterations in lung architecture result in reduced lung compliance, low volumes, and altered ventilation-perfusion matching. In the awake state, these abnormalities in function and structure combine to create hypoxemia, hyperventilation, and hypocapnia. Patients characteristically exhibit an increased breathing frequency and minute ventilation when awake at rest.[1]

Sleep Quality in Interstitial Lung Disease

Several studies have shown significant respiratory abnormalities during sleep.[2] Oxyhemoglobin desaturations (dSATs) are frequent, especially during rapid eye movement (REM) sleep when the degree of hypoventilation[2] and the degree of dSAT correlate with both the daytime oxygenation and the severity of the interstitial abnormality.[3] During non-REM (NREM) sleep in hypoxemic patients with ILD, initial reports described the maintenance of the increased respiratory frequency seen during wakefulness.[4] Compensatory increases in the hypoxic ventilatory drive confounded the results, however, because patients had diurnal hypoxemia. When the hypoxic ventilatory drive was eliminated with supplemental oxygen, patients with ILD had significantly reduced ventilation and respiratory frequency in slow wave sleep compared with the values observed during wakefulness. The increased drive to breathe during wakefulness may be behaviorally dependent on cortical perception of afferent information from the respiratory system, which disappears in NREM sleep.[5]

Few studies have looked critically or systematically at sleep quality in ILD. In one study of 37 patients, polysomnograms revealed that total sleep time, time spent in NREM sleep stage 3 and 4, and in REM sleep were decreased. The patients had poor sleep efficiency and they spent more time in wakefulness after sleep onset.[3] Other investigators described disrupted sleep, with more arousals, sleep-stage changes, and sleep fragmentation when compared with normal subjects.[2,4] Patients with an oxyhemoglobin

Mayo Sleep Disorders Center, 4500 San Pablo Road, Jacksonville, FL 32224, USA
E-mail address: kaplan.joseph@mayo.edu

Sleep Med Clin 3 (2008) 517–524
doi:10.1016/j.jsmc.2008.07.004
1556-407X/08/$ – see front matter

saturation (SAT) of less than 90% had more disrupted sleep than did those with SATs above 90%. Sleep stages were also redistributed, with a marked increase in stage 1 and a reduction in REM sleep.[2,4]

Sleep-Related Respiratory Abnormalities in Interstitial Lung Disease

Nocturnal hypoxemia represents the most characteristic gas exchange abnormality in patients with ILD. Clark and colleagues[6] evaluated the impact of nocturnal hypoxemia on quality of life in 48 patients with a mean SAT of 92.5%. The median number of dips greater than 4% per hour was of 2.3 per hour. Daytime SAT predicted mean overnight SAT but the percentage of the predicted forced vital capacity did not. Nocturnal hypoxemia was associated with decreased energy levels and impaired daytime social and physical functioning. These effects were independent of the forced vital capacity.

TREATMENT

Therapy usually involves the use of supplemental oxygen but the impact on sleep quality is variable. Patients with ILD who had acclimatized to moderate altitude (2240 m) and who had a mean SAT of 82.3% failed to demonstrate a change in sleep efficiency or arousals with the addition of oxygen therapy even though the mean SAT increased to 94.8%. Oxygen substantially decreased heart rate and respiratory rate, but did not normalize the respiratory rate.[7]

EXTRAPULMONARY RESTRICTION

Several disease states are associated with extrapulmonary restriction:

> Kyphoscoliosis
> Chest wall deformity
> Paralytic poliomyelitis
> Pott's disease
> Ankylosing spondylitis
> Marfan syndrome
> Mucopolyaccharidoses

Pure kyphosis without scoliosis may be seen in osteoporosis of the spine but is rarely associated with the same degree of pulmonary impairment seen in kyphoscoliosis.[8]

Kyphoscoliosis represents the prototype for restrictive extrapulmonary (chest cage) disorders. The condition is characterized by lateral curvature of the spine accompanied by rotation of the vertebrae. Most cases are idiopathic. Others develop as the result of poliomyelitis, neurofibromatosis,

tuberculosis, spondylitis and ankylosing spondylitis, or Marfan syndrome. Females outnumber males with the diagnosis. Respiratory failure develops in those patients who have reached greater than 100 degrees of spinal curvature measured by the Cobb technique.[9]

Abnormal lung mechanics predominate the abnormal physiology of patients with kyphoscoliosis. Shallow breathing develops as a defense mechanism designed to counteract the markedly increased work of breathing. The lower tidal volume results in increased dead space ventilation. Reduced lung volumes are associated with the closure of small airways, abnormal distribution of inspired air, and atelectasis, which all contribute to ventilation-perfusion mismatch and resultant hypoxemia. Low functional residual capacity results in low oxygen stores and in turn puts the patient at risk for more rapid dSAT with any level of sleep-disordered breathing.

Patients with kyphoscoliosis also develop problems with control of breathing. Two potential mechanisms may be operative. In patients with a history of poliomyelitis, the disease affects the medullary centers in addition to the respiratory muscles. In others, an acquired blunting of the ventilatory response to hypercapnia probably results from the high mechanical load much like the response seen in obesity.[10,11]

Clinical Features

As kyphoscoliosis progresses, patients develop several sequelae of chronic hypoventilation and hypoxemia including erthrocytosis, pulmonary hypertension, and cor pulmonale. Dyspnea may be lacking even in the face of hypoxemia and hypercapnia.

Sleep Quality in Kyphoscoliosis

Several investigators have identified disturbed nocturnal sleep and excessive daytime sleepiness in patients with kyphoscoliosis. Initial studies revealed lighter, more fragmented sleep with increased stage one and reduced stage 2 sleep.[12,13] In a more recent study, baseline polysomnograms showed fragmented sleep with low percentages of deep NREM sleep and REM sleep, and respiratory patterns characterized by very high breathing frequencies coinciding with significant dSATs.[14]

Sleep-Related Ventilatory and Gas Exchange Abnormalities

Patients with kyphoscoliosis exhibit characteristic ventilatory and gas exchange abnormalities during sleep. During REM sleep, intercostal and accessory muscles are inhibited.[15] REM-associated loss of muscle tone in the intercostal and accessory muscles results in a characteristic REM-only pattern of oxyhemoglobin dSAT (**Fig. 1**). Hypoxemia to levels less than 60% has been reported.[16]

Guilleminault and colleagues[12] were among the first to recognize sleep-disordered breathing in kyphoscoliosis. They described five patients with Cobb angles of 100, 110, 90, 110, and 115 (mean degree of spinal deformity = 105 degrees). All patients had evidence of mild to moderately severe restrictive ventilatory defects. All were found to have apneic events during sleep associated with dSAT. Some disordered-breathing events were obstructive in nature. The severity of the disordered breathing and dSAT correlated with both the subjective complaints of disturbed sleep and with cardiac failure. Sinus arrhythmia was seen in all patients and in most cases was the result of an arousal-associated tachycardia as respiratory events were terminated.

Patients frequently experience nocturnal and morning headache probably related to hypercapnia-mediated cerebral vasodilation. Awake carbon dioxide (CO_2) correlates with the nocturnal rise in CO_2.[17,18] Cheyne-Stokes respiratory pattern (with or without apneas), severe central apneas, and hypoventilation, especially in REM sleep, are common in this population.[13]

Treatment

Before the advent of nocturnal respiratory support, attempts to treat patients with kyphoscoliosis and chronic respiratory failure were largely unsuccessful. Daytime interventions including supplementary oxygen, digoxin, diuretics, tracheostomy, and intermittent positive pressure ventilation with inspired pressures of 25 cm H_2O four times a day failed in one small study.[19]

Drug therapy with protriptyline (10–20 mg at bedtime) aimed at suppressing REM sleep showed some promise.[20] In a trial involving eight patients, REM sleep fell from 22% to 12%. The total time spent at arterial oxygen SAT of less than 80% decreased and the magnitude of the fall correlated with the reduction in REM sleep. There was also a reduction in the maximum (CO_2) tension reached during the night. The arterial

oxygen tension measured diurnally increased from a median of 60 mm Hg to 67.5 mm Hg, but the CO_2 tension and base excess were unchanged. Anticholinergic side effects were experienced by most patients but did not limit treatment.[20] No other respiratory stimulants (progesterone, acetazolamide) have been systematically tested in this population.

The advent of nocturnal ventilatory support proved to be the first effective approach to patients with kyphoscoliosis who exhibit signs of chronic alveolar hypoventilation. **Table 1** summarizes much of the available data on the use of nocturnal intermittent positive pressure ventilation (NIPPV) for treatment of extrapulmonary restrictive diseases. Almost universally, patients respond with improved nighttime and daytime gas exchange,[14,19,21–27] improved quality of sleep,[19,21,25] improved daytime function,[19,21,27–29] and a reduction of hospitalizations.[22,23,30] Ventilator mode and settings used are usually directed initially by patient comfort and then adjusted according to measurements of gas tensions during wakefulness and confirmed during sleep. Some investigators have used transcutaneous CO_2 monitors to guide the level of nocturnal ventilatory support.[24,27] A nasal mask is usually preferable to a full facemask or mouthpiece.[31]

Insufflation leak is common during NIPPV and is associated with patient-ventilator asynchrony, ineffective efforts, persistent hypercapnia, and frequent arousals from sleep.[32] In bench studies, pressure-targeted ventilators perform better in the face of leak than volume-cycled flow generators. In contrast, volume-cycled ventilators should be able to deliver a higher tidal volume in the face of high impedance to inflation, but may just cause more leak.[33] In a recent Cochrane review, Annane and colleagues[34] recommended additional studies to compare the different types and modes of ventilation.

There is debate about whether the therapeutic aim of NIPPV should be to reduce respiratory muscle effort or to reverse nocturnal hypoventilation. When goals are not initially met, increasing support may be worthwhile. Tuggey and colleagues[35] provided increasing pressure support to several groups of patients in respiratory failure. Increased

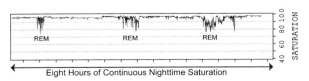

Fig. 1. Eight hours of continuous oximetry in a patient with kyphoscoliosis demonstrating REM-associated oxyhemoglobin desaturation.

Table 1
Summary of literature assessing the effectiveness of nocturnal intermittent positive pressure ventilation in patients with chest wall deformity

Studies	No. of Patients	Patient Characteristics	Type of Therapy	Duration of Therapy	Outcome
Hoeppner et al[19]	4	Severe kyphoscoliosis	NIPPV by tracheostomy	3.4 y	Resolution of right heart failure; Improved daytime blood gas levels; Decreased dyspnea; Improved sleep quality; Improved lung volumes; Decreased hemoglobin levels
Ellis et al[21]	5	Severe kyphoscoliosis; Mean age 34.4; Mean VC 0.97 ± 0.5	Nasal NIPPV	3 mo	Maintenance of Sao_2 and reduced $Tcco_2$; Improved daytime blood gas levels; Increased respiratory muscle strength; Increased length and quality of rapid eye movement sleep; Decreased daytime sleepiness and dyspnea
Hill et al[28]	6	Restrictive thoracic disease in chronic respiratory failure withdrawn for 1 week after 2 months on volume ventilators	Bilevel positive airway pressure	2 mo	Bilevel treatment ameliorated nocturnal hypoventilation and daytime symptoms; No change in pulmonary function, respiratory muscle strength, or blood gases
Jackson et al[30]	25	10 kyphoscoliosis; 8 thoracoplasty; 7 neuromuscular disease; Mean VC 30%	Nocturnal cuirass-assisted ventilation	5 y	Decreased hospitalizations
Leger et al[22]	105	Mean age 57; Mean VC 33%	Nasal NIPPV	1–2 y	Decreased number of hospitalizations; Improved daytime blood gas levels
Zaccaria et al[23]	13 stable13 recent episode of respiratory failure	Kyphoscoliosis in chronic respiratory failure	Nasal NIPPV (stable patients) or intermittent positive pressure ventilation by tracheostomy (recent episode of respiratory failure)	1 y	Improved daytime blood gas levels; Reduced hospital days

Study	N	Condition	Intervention	Duration	Results
Piper and Sullivan[24]	14	5 scoliosis, 5 muscle disease, 3 poliomyelitis	Nasal ventilation-volume ventilator (13 patients), pressure-cycled (one patient)	6 mo	Improved daytime blood gas levels; Increased respiratory muscle strength
Schlenker et al[25]	5	Kyphoscoliosis in chronic respiratory failure	NIPPV	6 mo	Increased respiratory muscle strength; Improved daytime blood gas levels; Increased total sleep time; Decreased pulmonary artery pressure
Ergun et al[26]	12	Restrictive thoracic disease in chronic respiratory failure	Daytime bilevel positive airway pressure 2 h/d	15 d	Decreased dyspnea; Improved daytime blood gas levels; Increased forced vital capacity; Increased 6-min walk
Gonzales et al[27]	16	Severe kyphoscoliosis Mean age 57.31 ± 8.46 Mean Cobb 97.64 ± 19.72	Nasal NIPPV with volume-cycled and pressure-cycled ventilator	36 mo	Improved daytime blood gas levels, respiratory muscle performance, and hypoventilation-based symptoms; No change in sleep architecture; No differences in breathing pattern or ventilatory drive
Fuschillo et al[29]	6	Severe kyphoscoliosis Nocturnal and exercise-induced desaturation	Nasal NIPPV Volume ventilator in assist-control mode	7 d	Improved nocturnal saturation; Improved exercise capacity; No change in spirometry, daytime blood gases, exercise desaturation
Laserna et al[14]	10	Kyphoscoliosis in chronic respiratory failure	Nasal NIPPV with volume-cycled compared with and pressure-cycled ventilator (bilevel positive airway pressure)	1 mo	Symptoms and daytime blood gases improved; Nocturnal oxygenation improved; Bilevel pressure cycled units as good as volume-cycled ventilators and better tolerated

Abbreviations: NIPPV, nocturnal intermittent positive pressure ventilation; VC, vital capacity.

pressure did result in more leaks, but an increase in minute ventilation was still achieved. In the cohort that had chest wall disease, the mean tolerated inspiratory pressure was 24 cm H_2O (8–40) and the set tidal volume was 9.6 mL/kg. Measures of respiratory effort were reduced at all levels regardless of whether ventilation was pressure or volume targeted. The findings support increasing the inspiratory pressure until therapeutic goals are reached tolerating any associated mask leak.

For NIPPV to be effective in sleep, a seal must be naturally created by the soft palate falling against the tongue to prevent excessive insufflation leakage and subsequent dSAT. Bach and Alba[31] reported the types of insufflation leakage and dSAT in 36 patients with chronic alveolar hypoventilation using NIPPV. Some patients showed a passive mechanical seal but most demonstrated a sawtooth pattern of dSATs throughout the night associated with arousal-mediated tongue and pharyngeal movements attempting to decrease leakage. In a few patients, the leak was so severe that patients were forced to switch to other noninvasive methods or tracheostomy-facilitated ventilatory assistance.

In a follow-up study looking specifically at patients with kyphoscoliosis and chronic alveolar hypoventilation, Bach and colleagues[36] evaluated sleep and air leakage with polysomnograms in kyphoscoliotic individuals who were using NIPPV.

The highest percentage of dSATs per unit time occurred during REM sleep despite fewer problems with insufflation leak during REM sleep. As seen in obstructive sleep apnea, dSATs and arousals were more common in stages 1, 2, and REM sleep and were reduced in slow wave sleep. With the use of NIPPV, improvements in symptoms, blood gases, and nocturnal dSATs were noted despite polysomnographically observed sleep disruption and sleep stage changes. Arousals and stage changes were associated with frequent transient dSATs and massive insufflation leakage. The authors identified specific oromotor activity, initiated centrally to decrease or eliminate leakage and normalize SAT. They concluded that the effectiveness of NIPPV was dependent in part on central-mediated compensatory muscular activity.

Several investigators have evaluated survival in patients with kyphoscoliosis and respiratory failure treated with NIPPV. **Table 2** summarizes the results. Buyse and colleagues[37] demonstrated better survival in kyphoscoliotic patients treated with NIPPV combined with long-term oxygen therapy. Gustafson and colleagues[38] evaluated Swedish patients with nonparalytic (not related to neuromuscular disease) kyphoscoliosis and found a significant survival advantage in the patients who received home mechanical ventilation compared with long-term oxygen therapy alone. In a group of patients with chest wall deformity from

Table 2
Summary of literature assessing survival in patients with chest wall deformity treated with nocturnal intermittent positive pressure ventilation

Studies	Study Type	Patient Characteristics	Type of Therapy (No. of Patients)	Duration of Therapy	Outcome
Buyse et al[37]	Retrospective	Kyphoscoliosis with chronic respiratory insufficiency	Long-term oxygen (15) NIPPV (18)	12 y	Improved 1-year survival for NIPPV group (100% versus 66%)
Gustafson et al[38]	Prospective	Nonparalytic kyphoscoliosis	Long-term oxygen (144) Home mechanical ventilation (100)	8 y	HMV associated with better survival than LTOT alone
Jäger et al[39]	Prospective	Chest wall deformity from tuberculosis	Long-term oxygen (103) Home mechanical ventilation (85)	8 y	Threefold better survival with home mechanical ventilation (adjusted for confounding variables)

Abbreviations: HMV, home mechanical ventilation; LTOT, long-term oxygen therapy.

tuberculosis, Jäger and colleagues[39] found that patients treated with home mechanical ventilation (with or without oxygen) had an almost threefold-better survival than patients treated with long-term oxygen alone even after adjustments for age, gender, concomitant respiratory disease, blood gas tensions, and vital capacity.

Budweiser and colleagues[40] evaluated the predictors of survival in patients with restrictive pulmonary disease in respiratory failure treated with noninvasive home ventilation. Patients were assessed before initiation of NIPPV and every 6 months over a period of 10 years. By univariate analysis, higher nighttime arterial CO_2 tensions, base excess, and lower hemoglobin at baseline predicted poor survival. Multivariate analysis identified nighttime arterial CO_2 tension as the only independent predictor of survival.

SUMMARY

In patients with restrictive ventilatory disease, sleep-associated hypoventilation often results in daytime functional sequelae and contributes to the poor prognosis seen in these patients. Although supplemental oxygen therapy may alleviate the nocturnal hypoxemia, NIPPV with or without oxygen seems to improve daytime function and offers a survival advantage in severe disease.

REFERENCES

1. Lourenco RV, Turino GM, Davidson LA, et al. The regulation of ventilation in diffuse pulmonary fibrosis. Am J Med 1965;38:199–216.
2. Bye PT, Issa F, Berthon-Jones M, et al. Studies of oxygenation during sleep in patients with interstitial lung disease. Am Rev Respir Dis 1984;129(1):27–32.
3. Aydoǎdu M, Ciftci B, Firat Güven S, et al. [Assessment of sleep with polysomnography in patients with interstitial lung disease]. Tuberk Toraks 2006;54(3):213–21 [in Turkish].
4. Perez-Padilla R, West P, Lertzman M, et al. Breathing during sleep in patients with interstitial lung disease. Am Rev Respir Dis 1985;132(2):224–9.
5. Shea SA, Winning AJ, McKenzie E, et al. Does the abnormal pattern of breathing in patients with interstitial lung disease persist in deep non-rapid eye movement sleep? Am Rev Respir Dis 1989;139(3):653–8.
6. Clark M, Cooper B, Singh S, et al. A survey of nocturnal hypoxaemia and health related quality of life in patients with cryptogenic fibrosing alveolitis. Thorax 2001;56(6):482–6.
7. Vazquez JC, Perez-Padilla R. Effect of oxygen on sleep and breathing in patients with interstitial lung disease at moderate altitude. Respiration 2001;68(6):584–9.
8. Leech JA, Dulberg C, Kellie S, et al. Relationship of lung functions to severity of osteoporosis in women. Am Rev Respir Dis 1990;141(1):68–71.
9. Cobb JR. Outline for the study of scoliosis. In: Edwards JW, editor. American Academy of orthopedic surgeons. Instructional course lectures. Ann Arbor (MI): The Academy; 1984. p. 261–75.
10. Bergofsky EH, Turinto GM, Fishman AP. Cardiorespiratory failure in kyphoscoliosis. Medicine (Baltimore) 1959;38:263–317.
11. Kafer ER. Respiratory function in paralytic scoliosis. Am Rev Respir Dis 1974;110(4):450–7.
12. Guilleminault C, Kurland G, Winkle R, et al. Severe kyphoscoliosis, breathing, and sleep: the Quasimodo syndrome during sleep. Chest 1981;79(6):626–30.
13. Mezon BL, West P, Israels J, et al. Sleep breathing abnormalities in kyphoscoliosis. Am Rev Respir Dis 1980;122(4):617–21.
14. Laserna E, Barrot E, Beiztegui A, et al. [Non-invasive ventilation in kyphoscoliosis: a comparison of a volumetric ventilator and a BIPAP support pressure device]. Arch Bronconeumol 2003;39(1):13–8.
15. Duron B, Marlot D. Intercostal and diaphragmatic electric activity during wakefulness and sleep in normal unrestrained adult cat. Sleep 1980;3(3–4):269–80.
16. Midgren B. Oxygen desaturation during sleep as a function of the underlying respiratory disease. Am Rev Respir Dis 1990;141(1):43–6.
17. Sawicka EH, Branthwaite MA. Respiration during sleep in kyphoscoliosis. Thorax 1987;42(10):801–8.
18. Midgren B, Hansson L. Changes in transcutaneous PCO_2 with sleep in normal subjects and in patients with chronic respiratory diseases. Eur J Respir Dis 1987;71(5):388–94.
19. Hoeppner VH, Cockcroft DW, Dosman JA, et al. Night-time ventilation improves respiratory failure in secondary kyphoscoliosis. Am Rev Respir Dis 1984;129(2):240–3.
20. Simonds AK, Parker RA, Branthwaite MA. Effects of protriptyline on sleep-related disturbances of breathing in restrictive chest wall disease. Thorax 1986;41:586–90.
21. Ellis ER, Grunstein RR, Chan S, et al. Noninvasive ventilatory support during sleep improves respiratory failure in kyphoscoliosis. Chest 1988;94(4):811–5.
22. Leger P, Bedicam JM, Cornette A, et al. Nasal intermittent positive pressure ventilation: long-term follow-up in patients with severe chronic respiratory insufficiency. Chest 1994;105(1):100–5.

23. Zaccaria S, Ioli F, Lusuardi M, et al. Long-term nocturnal mechanical ventilation in patients with kyphoscoliosis. Monaldi Arch Chest Dis 1995;50(6):433–7.

24. Piper AJ, Sullivan CE. Effects of long-term nocturnal nasal ventilation on spontaneous breathing during sleep in neuromuscular and chest wall disorders. Eur Respir J 1996;9:1515–22.

25. Schlenker E, Feldmeyer F, Hoster M, et al. Effect of noninvasive ventilation on pulmonary artery pressure in patients with severe kyphoscoliosis. Med Klin (Munich) 1997;92(Suppl 1):40–4.

26. Ergün P, Aydin G, Turay UY, et al. Short-term effect of nasal intermittent positive pressure ventilation in patients with restrictive thoracic disease. Respiration 2002;69(4):303–8.

27. Gonzales C, Ferris G, Diaz J, et al. Kyphoscoliotic ventilatory insufficiency: effects of long-term intermittent positive-pressure ventilation. Chest 2003; 124(3):857–62.

28. Hill NS, Eveloff SE, Carlisle CC, et al. Efficacy of nocturnal ventilation in patients with restrictive thoracic disease. Am Rev Respir Dis 1992;145(2 Pt 1): 365–71.

29. Fuschillo S, De Felice A, Gaudiosi C, et al. Nocturnal mechanical ventilation improves exercise capacity in kyphoscoliotic patients with respiratory impairment. Monaldi Arch Chest Dis 2003;59(4):267–8.

30. Jackson M, Kinnear W, King M, et al. The effects of five years of nocturnal cuirass-assistec ventilation of chest wall disease. Eur Respir J 1993;6(5):630–5.

31. Bach JR, Alba AS. Management of chronic alveolar hypoventilation by nasal ventilation. Chest 1990; 97(1):52–7.

32. Teschler H, Stampa J, Ragette R, et al. Effect of mouth leaks on effectiveness of nasal bilevel ventilatory assistance and sleep architecture. Eur Respir J 1999;14(6):1251–7.

33. Mehta S, McCool FD, Hill NS. Leak compensation in positive pressure ventilators: a lung model study. Eur Respir J 2001;17(2):259–67.

34. Annane D, Chevrolet JC, Chevret S, et al. Nocturnal mechanical ventilation for chronic hypoventilation in patients with neuromuscular and chest wall disorders. Cochrane Database Syst Rev 2000;2: CD001941.

35. Tuggey JM, Elliott MW. Titration of non-invasive positive pressure ventilation in chronic respiratory failure. Respir Med 2006;100(7):1262–9 [Epub 2005 Nov 28].

36. Bach JR, Robert D, Leger P, et al. Sleep fragmentation in kyphoscoliotic individuals with alveolar hypoventilation treated NIPPV. Chest 1995;107(6): 1552–8.

37. Buyse B, Meersseman W, Demedts M. Treatment of chronic respiratory failure in kyphoscoliosis: oxygen or ventilation. Eur Respir J 2003;22(3):525–8.

38. Gustafson T, Franklin KA, Midgren B, et al. Survival of patients with kyphoscoliosis receiving mechanical ventilation or oxygen at home. Chest 2006;130(6): 1828–33.

39. Jäger L, Franklin KA, Midgren B, et al. Increased survival with mechanical ventilation in posttuberculosis patients with the combination of respiratory failure and chest wall deformity. Chest 2008;133(1): 156–60.

40. Budweiser S, Mürbeth RE, Jörres RA, et al. Predictors of long-term survival in patients with restrictive thoracic disorders and chronic respiratory failure undergoing non-invasive home ventilation. Respirology 2007;12(4):551–9 l.

Obesity Hypoventilation Syndrome

Meena Khan, MD, Karen L. Wood, MD, Nitin Y. Bhatt, MD*

KEYWORDS

- Obesity • Hypovenitilation • Sleep apnea

Obesity is a growing epidemic. Between 1986 and 2000, the obese population in the United States doubled.[1,2] Childhood obesity is also increasing. In the United States, the prevalence of obesity in children ages 5 to 12 tripled from 1960 to 2000.[3] Obesity is associated with a variety of health problems, including cardiovascular disease, hypertension, stroke, diabetes type II, dyslipidemia, cancer, and joint disease.[1,4] Obesity is also associated with an increased risk of early death, particularly in people who do not have significant health problems or tobacco use.[5] This trend spans all ages, including the elderly.[5] Among the diseases prevalent in this population is obesity hypoventilation syndrome (OHS). This article addresses OHS, its prevalence, clinical implications, pathophysiology, and treatment.

DEFINITION AND PHYSIOLOGY

The first descriptions of OHS go back to at least 1956.[6,7] These patients were clinically described as obese with hypersomnolence and associated periodic breathing, cyanosis, right ventricular hypertrophy, cor pulmonale, and secondary polycythemia.[8] This constellation of symptoms was termed *Pickwickian syndrome* after Charles Dickens' description of Joe, "a fat red faced boy in a state of solmnolency" in *The Pickwick Papers*.[9] Since then, the term *obesity hypoventilation* has been used to describe such patients and represents one type of sleep hypoventilation syndrome. According to the American Academy of Sleep Medicine's *International Classification of Sleep Disorders*, which categorizes sleep-related hypoventilation syndromes based on etiology, such disorders may be idiopathic in origin or they may be

due to pulmonary parenchymal or vascular pathology, lower airway obstruction, or neuromuscular and chest wall disorders. This last group, where obesity is the only identifiable cause of hypoventilation, includes OHS.[10]

The diagnostic criteria for sleep hypoventilation syndrome (**Box 1**) include the presence of clinical symptoms, an increase in $Paco_2$ of 10 mm Hg in sleep compared with supine wake state, or a greater than 10% desaturation during sleep not related to upper airway obstruction.[11] The hypoventilation is considered severe if the oxygen saturation during sleep is less than 85% for more than 50% of the sleep time or if signs of cor pulmonale or biventricular heart failure are present.[11] Obesity hypoventilation is a combination of obesity (defined as a body mass index [BMI (kg/m^2)] $\geq$ 30), unexplained daytime hypercapnia ($Paco_2 \geq$ 45 mm Hg), and sleep-disordered breathing.[12,13] The sleep-disordered breathing can be either obstructive sleep apnea (OSA) or sleep hypoventilation and tends to occur in those with morbid obesity (BMI $\geq$ 35).[11–13]

PREVALENCE

A recent review summarized nine studies with over 3000 patients and described the prevalence of OHS in patients with OSA as ranging from 10% to 20%.[13] A recent study looked at the percentage of OSA patients with OHS retrospectively and prospectively.[14] The retrospective arm had 180 patients and showed that 30% of OSA patients have OHS (defined as BMI > 30 and $Paco_2$ > 45 mm Hg). The prospective arm had 410 patients and showed a 20% prevalence of OHS.[14] Nowbar and colleagues[15] prospectively evaluated obese

Division of Pulmonary, Allergy, Critical Care, and Sleep Medicine, The Ohio State University, 201 Davis Heart and Lung Institute, 473 West 12th Avenue, Columbus, OH 43210, USA
* Corresponding author.
E-mail address: nitin.bhatt@osumc.edu (N.Y. Bhatt).

Sleep Med Clin 3 (2008) 525–539
doi:10.1016/j.jsmc.2008.08.001
1556-407X/08/$ – see front matter © 2008 Elsevier Inc. All rights reserved.

> **Box 1**
> **Diagnostic criteria for sleep hypoventilation syndrome**
>
> One or more of the following:
> Cor pulmonale
> Pulmonary hypertension
> Hypersomnia not otherwise explained
> Erythrocytosis
> Wake hypercapnia
> And one or more of the following:
> Increase in $Paco_2$ during sleep of more than 10 mm Hg from supine awake
> Oxygen desaturation in sleep not explained by apnea or hypopnea

patients (BMI $\geq$ 35) admitted to the hospital in an attempt to determine the percentage of patients meeting the criteria for OHS versus simple obesity. Of all patients admitted to the hospital, 6% had a BMI of 35 or more and, after excluding patients with other causes of hypoventilation or lung disease, 31% of the remaining patients had unexplained hypercapnia. Of those patients that met criteria for OHS, only 23% were given a diagnosis of OHS. Of these patients, only 13% had treatment of OHS included on their discharge instructions.[15] Therefore, OHS seems to be underrecognized and undertreated.

CLINICAL PRESENTATION AND PROGNOSIS

Those with OHS can have a characteristic constellation of symptoms and physical examination findings. The central symptoms are due to elevated $Paco_2$ and consist of cognitive impairment, hypersomnolence during the day, and morning headache.[15–18] There is also chronic hypoxemia during the wake state that leads to stigmata of pulmonary hypertension, cor pulmonale, erythrocytosis, and respiratory failure.[8,16,19,20] Sleep-disordered breathing can present with symptoms of fragmented sleep, loud snoring, choking, and gasping during sleep. Dependent peripheral edema, dyspnea, and orthopnea are also common.[8,13,16]

These patients may also have characteristic laboratory findings. Mokhlesi and colleagues[13] recently summarized the demographic, physical, and laboratory characteristics of patients with OHS reported in the literature (**Table 1**). These patients tended to be male and morbidly obese, with hypercapnia and hypoxemia, but a normal pH.

Nowbar and colleagues[15] found that the Pao_2 was significantly lower and serum bicarbonate was significantly higher in OHS patients compared with those with simple obesity. Also, significantly more patients with OHS had erythrocytosis (hemoglobin > 16.3 g/dL).[15] The above data show a trend of markedly abnormal arterial blood gases in terms of the degree of hypercapnia and hypoxemia in OHS patients, as well as an elevated serum bicarbonate and erythrocytosis.

OHS patient have been shown to have a higher morbidity and mortality, decreased quality of life, and an increased use of health care resources.[17,21] In 1974, Miller and Granada[20] reported on 10 patients followed over 5 years who had extreme obesity (weight 250–400 lb),

Table 1
Clinical features of patients with OHS

Variables	Mean Values (Range)[a]
Age (y)	52 (42–61)
Male gender (%)	66 (49–60)
BMI (kg/m^2)	44 (35–56)
Neck circumference (cm)	46.5 (45–47)
pH	7.38 (7.34–7.40)
$Paco_2$ (mm Hg)	52 (47–61)
Pao_2 (mm Hg)	60 (46–74)
Serum bicarbonate (mEq/L)	32 (31–33)
Haemoglobin (g/dL)	15
Apnea-hypopnea index	66 (20–100)
SaO_2 nadir during sleep (%)	65 (59–76)
Percentage of TST with SaO_2 < 90%	50 (46–56)
FVC (% predicted)	73 (57–102)
FEV_1 (% of predicted)	67 (53–92)
FEV_1/FVC ratio	77 (74–88)
MRC dyspnea class 3 and 4 (%)	69
Epworth Sleepiness Scale score	14 (12–16)
CPAP (cm H_2O) (n = 86)	14
Bi-level PAP (cm H_2O) (n = 55)	18/9

Abbreviations: CPAP, continuous positive air pressure; FEV_1, forced expiratory volume in 1 second; FVC, forced vital capacity; MRC, Medical Research Council; PAP, positive air pressure; SaO_2, arterial oxygen saturation; TST, total sleep time.
[a] Values for 631 patients with OHS.
From Mokhlesi B, Tulaimat A. Recent advances in obesity hypoventilation syndrome. Chest 2007;132(4):1322–36; with permission.

hypercapnia, and mental obtundation. Seven of the 10 died in the hospital—3 from respiratory failure, 3 from pulmonary embolism, and 1 from acute renal failure.[20] In 1970, MacGregor and colleagues[8] described the outcomes of 22 patients with OHS. Seven of them died (~31%), 5 from sudden death.[8] Autopsies were performed on all 7. No cause was stated on 3, 1 had myocardial infarction, 1 had pulmonary emboli, and 1 had a bleeding diathesis that was unrelated to OHS.[8] Nowbar and colleagues[15] reported that, at 18 months after hospital discharge, patients who met the criteria for OHS (BMI $\geq$ 35 and unexplained hypercapnia while awake with the P_{CO_2} $\geq$ 43 mm Hg) had a higher death rate than patients with obesity alone (23% vs. 9%) with a relative risk of death that is fourfold higher for OHS patients. Finally, OHS patients who refused treatment with noninvasive ventilation, had a mortality rate of 46% over an average follow-up period of 50 months, although the causes of death were not always known.[22]

Patients with OHS also suffer from other comorbid conditions. OHS patients are more likely to be diagnosed with congestive heart failure, hypertension, diabetes, angina, osteoarthritis, cor pulmonale, and hypothyroidism compared with the general population.[8,21] Compared to the obese population, OHS patients are more likely to be diagnosed with congestive heart failure, angina, and cor pulmonale.[21] They are also more likely to have pulmonary hypertension (defined as a mean pulmonary artery pressure > 20 mm Hg) and to have the lowest desaturations during sleep when compared with patients with OSA alone or in combination with chronic obstructive pulmonary disease.[23] If there is concomitant sleep apnea, OHS patients tend to have a higher respiratory disturbance index.[24] Comparing OHS patients to obese patients or those with OSA alone revealed that OHS patients have more hypercapnia and hypoxemia during the day, tend to be morbidly obese (BMI > 40), and have a higher incidence of pulmonary hypertension.[22-25]

Patients with OHS experience significant impairment in terms of quality-of-life measures. This includes poor memory and concentration, significant sleepiness, more frequent and longer hospital stays, more days in the intensive care unit, more invasive procedures, and a higher need for long-term care at discharge.[15,17,21] A study in Japan looked at quality of life and sleepiness in OHS, OSA, and controls.[17] In terms of sleepiness and social functioning, OHS patients scored worse than age- and BMI-matched OSA patients.[17]

OHS patients also consume more health care resources than do simple obese patients or an average patient population.[21] OHS patients had more physician visits and claims on average than simple obesity patients and controls did. Furthermore, OHS patients were associated with higher costs compared with simple obesity patients and controls. Those with OHS have a high mortality rate as well as significant comorbidities that impair quality of life and result in high health care cost. Despite this, the diagnosis of OHS appears to be often overlooked, especially in the hospital setting when dealing with the other illnesses of these patients. It is important to be aware of this diagnosis to facilitate treatment and improve patient outcomes.

BENEFITS OF DIAGNOSIS AND TREATMENT

Treatment of OHS has been shown to improve the symptoms and quality of life and to reduce morbidity and mortality. In a retrospective analysis of OHS patients discharged from the hospital with home noninvasive ventilation as treatmen,[26] survival at year 1 was 97.1%, year 2 was 92%, and year 5 was 70.2%, which is higher compared with survival rate shown for similar, untreated patients in other studies.[8,15,20,22,26] Clinical symptoms, such as hypersomnia, peripheral edema, sleep fragmentation, and dyspnea, and quality of life have all been shown to improve with noninvasive ventilation. Additionally, improvements in arterial blood gas, pulmonary hemodynamics, and pulmonary function tests have also been demonstrated.[15,18,22,27,28] Sleepiness and quality of life improve significantly after only 4 to 6 months of treatment in both OSA and OHS.[17]

After treatment, hospital admissions and length of stay decreased significantly as well.[21] In fact, during the second year of treatment, OHS patients were no more likely to be hospitalized than simple obese patients or a control population.[21] Based on the reduction in the number of days hospitalized after initiating treatment in OHS patients, the net health care cost savings per patient were estimated at $3900 after 1 year of treatment and $4400 after year 2 and in each additional year.[21]

The diagnosis of OHS can have a significant impact on an individual patient and on the health care system as a whole. Patients with OHS have significant symptoms as well as comorbidities that impair quality of life and lead to increased morbidity and mortality. Treatment of OHS leads to improvement of the subjective complaints as well as improvements in objective measures. Survival and cost of health care also significantly improve with treatment. This evidence supports that recognition and treatment of this disease is imperative.

EVALUATION AND DIAGNOSIS

The diagnosis of OHS must be considered when evaluating and treating patients with obesity or with sleep-disordered breathing. In patients with OSA, several clinical factors have been shown to be suggestive of underlying OHS. These include serum bicarbonate, apnea-hypopnea index (AHI [events per hour]), and the lowest oxygen desaturations during sleep.[14] Specifically, 50% of patients with OSA (defined as AHI > 5) who had a serum bicarbonate of 27 mEq/L or more, had OHS, compared with 3% of those with a bicarbonate less than 27 mEq/L. A normal bicarbonate seemed to rule out OHS. Additionally, 76% of those with an AHI of 100 or more had OHS compared with 39% of those with an AHI of less than 100.[14] The investigators concluded that serum bicarbonate represents an effective screening measure for OHS.[13,14]

In patients with obesity, the diagnosis of OHS can be confirmed with an awake arterial blood gas showing a Pa_{CO_2} of 45 mm Hg or more. If hypercapnia is found, other causes of hypoventilation must be excluded. **Boxes 2** and **3** outline the differential diagnosis as well as the clinical evaluation of this patient population. The differential diagnosis of hypercapnia includes central nervous system–depressant drugs; obstructive lung disease; restrictive lung diseases, including such chest wall deformities as kyphoscoliosis; neuromuscular disease or interstitial lung disease; hypothyroidism; and congenital central hypoventilation syndrome.[13,19,29] A thorough neurologic examination, thyroid function testing, pulmonary function testing, and chest radiography should be performed to rule out other causes of the hypercapnia.[13,16,19,27] An overnight polysomnography should also be performed to evaluate for sleep-disordered breathing.[25] If a diagnosis of OHS is made, it is important to evaluate for pulmonary hypertension or erythrocytosis as these

---

Box 2
Differential diagnosis of hypercapnia

OHS

Central nervous system depressants: narcotics, alcohol, benzodiazepines

Obstructive airway disease

Chest wall deformities: kyphoscoliosis

Neuromuscular disease

Interstitial lung disease

Hypothyroidism

Congenital central hypoventilation syndrome

Box 3
Evaluation of OHS

Suspicion of OHS

Serum bicarbonate

Arterial blood gas

Evaluation of hypercapnia

Pulmonary function test

Chest radiograph

Thyroid function test

Neurologic examination

Assessment of severity of OHS

Echocardiogram

Complete blood cell count (to evaluate for erythrocytosis)

---

indicate more serious disease.[29] This evaluation includes an echocardiogram and complete blood cell count.[29]

PATHOGENESIS

The pathogenesis of OHS is not completely understood. A combination of morbid obesity, OSA, and alterations in leptin levels combine to affect respiratory function and promote the formation of severe hypoxemia and hypercapnia seen in this syndrome.

Effect of Obesity on Pulmonary Function and Ventilation

Obesity is associated with decreased compliance of the respiratory system as a result of decreases in both the lung and chest wall compliances.[30,31] This decreased compliance is attributed to the negative effects of the extra body mass around the chest and abdomen in obese patients. In addition, the distribution of weight influences respiratory system compliance. Sharp and colleagues[32] compared mass loading of the thorax and abdomen and found the biggest decrease in compliance was after abdominal mass loading. This is consistent with other studies demonstrating that lung volumes decrease because of elevated abdominal pressures in patients who are sedated and paralyzed.[33]

The mechanical effects of mass loading lead obese patients to breathe at lower lung volumes. In fact, the most noticeable and recognized pulmonary function testing abnormalities in obesity are drops in the expiratory reserve volume (ERV) and the functional residual capacity (FRC).[34] Even a small amount of weight gain can cause rapid drops in ERV and FRC. In people with a BMI of 30, the ERV is less than half the value than those with a BMI of 20.[35] These effects are accentuated in the supine position as both lung compliance and ERV decrease in the supine position in a linear relationship.[36] This positional drop in ERV has also been correlated with the decrease in Pa_{O_2} seen in morbidly obese patients in the supine position.[37]

Obesity has smaller but still potentially clinically significant effects on other measures of lung volumes. There is a modest negative correlation between obesity and total lung capacity, vital capacity, and the residual volume (**Fig. 1**).[35] The diffusing capacity is normal or slightly elevated in obesity, reflecting the relatively normal lung parenchyma and increased blood circulation through the lungs.[35,38] Obesity has also been linked with an increase in airway resistance,[39] likely due to narrowing and collapsibility of the upper airways by the mechanical load placed on the upper airway and thorax.[40]

This increased resistance, decreased respiratory compliance, and increased metabolic demands lead to an increased work of breathing in obese subjects.[41] Therefore, obesity is associated with an increased ventilatory drive.[42,43] Most obese patients are able to meet this increased demand and maintain eucapnia. In the normal state, Pa_{CO_2} is normally tightly controlled, so that minor changes in Pa_{CO_2} levels stimulate peripheral and central chemoreceptors to cause an increase in minute ventilation by changes in both tidal volume and respiratory frequency, the "hypercapnic respiratory drive." Simple eucapnic obesity is associated with a normal hypoxic ventilatory response, and a slightly abnormal (decreased) hypercapnic ventilatory response.[42] In comparison, patients with OHS have a decreased hypoxic and hypercapnic ventilatory drive.[44] This blunted response to hypercapnia and hypoxemia distinguish OHS from simple obesity. The result is that, in OHS, the minute ventilation falls below a range necessary to compensate for the metabolic demands and hypercapnia results.

The importance of obesity in the pathogenesis of OHS is highlighted by clinical data noting obese patients with increased restrictive lung disease have worse hypercapnia.[45,46] In support of this, weight loss by bariatric surgery improves hypercapnia, hypoxemia,[47] and ventilatory response to P_{CO_2}.[43] Interestingly, in response to treatment of OHS with noninvasive positive-pressure ventilation (NIPPV), ERV is one respiratory function parameter that increased and was seemingly independent of changes in BMI.[48]

Effects of Obstructive Sleep Apnea on Ventilation

Can OSA cause obese patients to be hypercapnic? There are conflicting data and no clear answer to this question. In one study of 219 patients who underwent hypercapnic ventilatory response testing and polysomnogram, the only variables that correlated with a decreased hypercapnic response were high daytime Pa_{CO_2} and older age in men, whereas in women an elevated BMI correlated with an increase in hypercapnic ventilatory response. There was no relationship between hypercapnic respiratory drive and OSA.[49] Increased apneic duration was correlated with hypercapnia in one study, but it included patients with chronic obstructive pulmonary disease.[50] Another study showed that the severity of OSA based on AHI

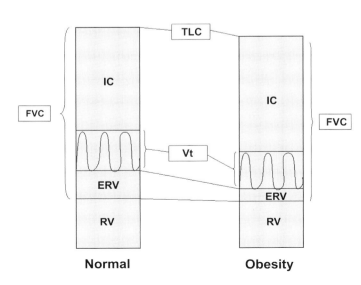

Normal   **Obesity**

Fig. 1. Comparison of lung volumes in obese and normal individuals. FVC, forced vital capacity; IC, inspiratory capacity; RV, residual volume; TLC, total lung capacity; Vt, tidal volume.

was associated with hypercapnia.[51] However, others have shown no relationship between AHI and hypercapnia.[45,52] It has been hypothesized that the sleep fragmentation and chronic hypoxia seen in OSA may lead to blunting of the respiratory drive and hypercapnia.[12] This is supported by studies that have correlated nocturnal desaturation (but not AHI) with hypercapnia.[45]

Another hypothesis to explain the link between OSA and hypercapnia attributes daytime hypercapnia and decreased sensitivity to elevated carbon dioxide levels to the repetitive episodes of acute hypercapnia that occurs after the apneas in OSA.[53,54] The effect of treatment of OSA on levels of daytime $Paco_2$ is another way to indirectly propose a relationship between OSA and hypercapnia. Studies have shown a reduction in daytime $Paco_2$ of around 7 mm Hg after starting continuous positive airway pressure (CPAP) therapy.[55–57] The effect of therapy on the hypercapnic ventilatory response in patients with OSA is more conflicting. While some studies have shown that there was improvement in hypercapnic ventilatory response[57,58] with CPAP therapy, others showed no improvement in hypercapnic ventilatory response in patients with OSA (not OHS) treated with CPAP compared with sham CPAP, although there was a reduction in the ventilatory response to hypoxia during treatment for 1 month.[59] CPAP has beneficial effects on the respiratory system with unloading of the respiratory muscles and may decrease carbon dioxide by those effects. However, studies looking at tracheostomy, which directly alleviates the upper airway obstruction, may provide better evidence of the effect of OSA on OHS. One interesting study followed eight hypercapnic patients (seven treated with tracheostomy, one with CPAP) successfully treated for OSA.[27] Four of the eight patients corrected their $Paco_2$ to normal levels after treatment of OSA, while four remained hypercapnic. The only differences between these two groups were that the patients that corrected their $Paco_2$ after treatment of sleep apnea had normal levels of ventilation while awake before the treatment, while the four that did not correct had low levels of ventilation while awake. Taken together, these studies would suggest that OSA may "tip the scales" in some people with a predisposition to OHS, but is unlikely to be the sole factor responsible for the development of hypercapnia and the OHS.

LEPTIN RESISTANCE—THE MISSING LINK?

Obesity and OSA can both cause changes in lung mechanics and ventilatory patterns that in combination may explain the hypercapnia seen in OHS.

However, many obese patients do not have OSA or hypercapnia and not all patients with OSA and obesity have OHS. The discovery of leptin, a recent and intriguing finding, may help to explain why some patients develop elevated $Paco_2$ levels while others are spared.

The obese (ob) gene encodes the protein leptin, which acts on the hypothalamus to cause satiety.[60–62] Leptin-deficient (ob/ob) mice are obese and have a rapid breathing pattern and a blunted ventilatory response to increasing levels of $Paco_2$.[63,64] They also have significantly higher levels of daytime $Paco_2$,[19] and therefore have many similarities with the OHS phenotype. Interestingly, leptin replacement in mice increases baseline awake minute ventilation (both tidal volume and respiratory frequency) as well as ventilation during sleep (rapid eye movement [REM] and non–REM in the leptin-deficient mouse C57BL/6J-Lep[ob]). This increase in ventilation was thought to be a result of a neurally mediated mechanism and not changes in metabolic rates.[19]

In humans, there have been rare cases of mutation in the leptin gene leading to leptin deficiency[65] and mutations in the leptin receptor gene resulting in markedly elevated serum leptin levels and leptin resistance.[66] Both of these mutations are associated with morbid obesity. However, carbon dioxide levels have not been reported in these families.

At first, it appeared a simple story with decreased leptin resulting in morbid obesity. However, there has been much conflicting data on the role of leptin. While leptin deficiency results in obesity, obesity (not related to genetic deficiency or receptor mutation) has also been associated with elevated levels of leptin in mice and humans.[67,68] It has been hypothesized that elevated leptin levels may be a compensatory mechanism by which obese subjects maintain normal levels of carbon dioxide, but resistance to leptin may develop. In obese patients, leptin levels correlate with BMI.[69] Elevated leptin levels are a better predictor of hypercapnia than percentage of body fat[70,71] and a recent evaluation of 245 patients (186 of whom underwent hypercapnic response testing) confirmed elevated leptin levels were a better predictor of decreased respiratory drive and a reduced ventilatory response to hypercapnia than percent body fat.[72] As has been shown in a mouse model of obesity, there is a resistance to transport of leptin across the blood-brain barrier.[73] In humans, an alteration in the serum–to–cerebrospinal fluid ratio of leptin has suggested impaired cerebrospinal fluid transport of leptin into the cerebrospinal fluid.[74,75] High-fat diets may also induce resistance to leptin.[76] Therefore, although the data are not conclusive, it has been hypothesized that in OHS there is leptin resistance leading to a "relative deficiency" and predisposing to hypercapnia and blunted respiratory response.

Treatment trials support that leptin may be important in the pathophysiology of OHS, but the data remain inconsistent. One trial showed NIPPV increased plasma leptin levels[58] while another reported decreased serum leptin levels after NIPPV.[77] Interestingly, the study by Redolfi and colleagues[58] compared six patients with OHS (without OSA, nocturnal hypoventilators) with six eucapnic obese patients and found OHS was associated with lower leptin levels that increased with NIPPV. Meanwhile, a study from Rapoport and colleagues[27] showed that patients with daytime hypoventilation did not improve after treatment of OSA with tracheostomy, but those with normal daytime ventilation and OSA did improve their hypercapnia. These studies demonstrate that perhaps there is a different pathophysiology associated with different OHS phenotypes (**Fig. 2**).

TREATMENT

The mechanisms behind OHS remain incompletely understood and the physiologic derangements seen with OHS are multifactorial in origin. These derangements include alterations in respiratory mechanics from obesity, central dysregulation of respiratory control, and sleep-disordered breathing. The mainstay of therapy for OHS is targeted at correction of hypoventilation and sleep-disordered breathing through positive airway pressure (PAP), such as continuous PAP (CPAP) or NIPPV, using bi-level PAP or noninvasive volume-cycled ventilation. Patients with OHS have underlying sleep-disordered breathing and this can be obstructive or, less commonly, central in nature.[23,78] The use of PAP for correction of OSA is well described and its role in OHS is becoming better understood.

A significant number of patients are diagnosed with OHS at the time of an episode of acute respiratory failure or may develop an acute decompensation of their chronic respiratory failure. CPAP and, more commonly, NIPPV have been shown to be beneficial in this acute setting, resulting in a decreased need for endotracheal intubation and improved mortality.[79–81] Improvement in arterial blood gas measures were seen within days and, in some cases, normalized within a month.[22,80] Similar benefits were also seen in the chronic presentation.[22,79,80,82–84] The use of bi-level PAP has also been shown to improve $Paco_2$, AHI, sleep architecture with increased slow wave sleep and increased REM sleep, and Epworth Sleepiness Scale score within a week of initiating therapy.[18] In these studies, up to 50% of patients treated with PAP may require supplemental nocturnal oxygen. Many eucapnic OSA patients who are intolerant of CPAP are treated with supplemental oxygen for nocturnal desaturation. The use of oxygen was compared with NIPPV in patients with restrictive chest wall disease due to obesity (OHS) or neuromuscular disease and kyphoscoliosis. Patients in each group received home oxygen for 2 weeks followed by home NIPPV with bi-level PAP or a volume-cycled ventilator for 2 weeks.[85] In the patients with OHS, the use of supplemental oxygen showed no improvement in clinical symptoms while NIPPV resulted in a decrease in dyspnea, morning headaches, and morning obtundation. Pao_2 was improved in both treatment groups. However, hypoventilation was only improved with NIPPV. Thus, supplemental oxygen alone appears not to be adequate therapy for patients with OHS.

PAP and NIPPV have both been associated with improvements in daytime hypercapnia and

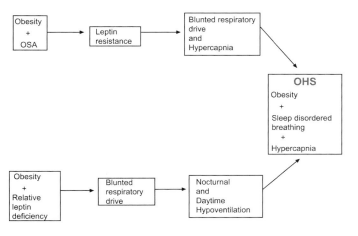

Fig. 2. Proposed pathways leading to the obesity hypoventilation syndrome.

hypoxemia.[56] This effect was quantified in a retrospective cohort analysis of 75 patients with OHS. Eighty percent were being treated with CPAP, 20% were on bi-level ventilation, and posttreatment evaluation occurred after at least 30 days of PAP therapy. Patients whose adherence to therapy (defined as more than 4.5 hours of PAP daily) had a Pa_{CO_2} decrease of 7.7 mm Hg in comparison to 2.4 mm Hg in those less adherent. The follow-up Pa_{CO_2} had normalized (< 45 mm Hg) in 34% of adherent patients as compared with only 17% of those with adherence below 4.5 hours. Similarly, adherent patients had an increase in Pa_{O_2} of 9.2 mm Hg compared with a 1.8-mm Hg increase in less adherent patients. No other variables contributed to this change in arterial blood gas measurements except use of PAP. The relationship between adherence and Pa_{CO_2} response was shown to plateau after 7 hours of daily use while Pa_{O_2} response to PAP therapy reached a plateau at approximately 4.5 hours.

As both CPAP and bi-level ventilation have been shown to be effective in the treatment of patients with OHS, the optimal approach to treatment remains to be determined. Only one study has directly compared CPAP to bi-level ventilatory support.[55] This prospective, randomized study included 36 OHS patients not being treated with PAP at the time of enrollment and not having signs of respiratory decompensation based on pH and P_{CO_2}. All patients underwent a baseline CPAP study and those who showed significant oxygen desaturation (< 80% continuously for > 10 minutes) in the absence of apnea, an acute rise in transcutaneous carbon dioxide of more than 10 mm Hg during REM sleep on CPAP, or an increase in afternoon-to-morning P_{CO_2} of greater than or equal to 10 mm Hg were deemed as CPAP failures, treated with bi-level ventilation and excluded from the study. Thirty-six patients were enrolled and equally allocated to the CPAP and bi-level groups. At 3 months, compliance with therapy was equivalent, averaging approximately 6 hours per night, and there were equal reductions in weight and daytime Pa_{CO_2} between the groups. Improvements in daytime oxygen saturation, serum bicarbonate, Epworth Sleepiness Scale score, and the Short Form 36 health survey score were also equal. The bi-level group did show a subjective improvement in terms of the Pittsburgh Sleep Quality Index, as well as a better performance on psychomotor vigilance testing. These results are likely not applicable to patients with ongoing nocturnal desaturation or hypoventilation while on CPAP. In fact, these investigators had previously shown that nonresponders to CPAP may require NIPPV during sleep.[80]

Thus, the appropriate approach to PAP titration remains to be determined. In most cases, CPAP is tried initially and titrated to eliminate obstructive events and signs of airflow limitation. CPAP in the range of 12 to 20 cm H_2O have generally been required.[80,84,86] In the presence of ongoing desaturation or inability to eliminate airflow limitation or patient intolerance of high CPAP pressures, bi-level ventilation has been initiated. In most studies, inspiratory positive airway pressures (IPAPs) ranged from 12 to 30 cm H_2O and expiratory positive airway pressures (EPAPs) ranged from 5 to 12 cm H_2O. In general, a difference of 8 to 10 cm H_2O between IPAP and EPAP was required.[22,26,58,87] For OHS patients without OSA, bi-level ventilation is recommended.

Despite the beneficial effects of PAP, treatment may not correct hypoxemia or hypercapnia in all patients with OHS. A significant number of patients may show ongoing nocturnal desaturation despite the correction of obstructive events with PAP. In a study examining the response to 1 night of CPAP in eucapnic OSA patients compared with those with OHS, the use of CPAP was associated with a significant improvement in AHI, reduction in arousals, and improved REM sleep time. However, 43% of the patients with OHS had ongoing nocturnal desaturation despite a significant improvement in AHI from baseline. These patients did have a higher BMI and an increased REM AHI. However, they were otherwise similar in terms of pulmonary function and arterial blood gases to the remainder of the OHS patients whose nocturnal desaturation corrected with CPAP.[86] The response to hypercapnia may also be incomplete. Eight of the 34 patients who used PAP for at least 4.5 hours per day did not show a significant improvement in their Pa_{CO_2}, defined as a decrease in Pa_{CO_2} of less than 4 mm Hg. These nonresponders had a lower AHI compared with responders, but were otherwise similar in age, race, gender, BMI, AHI, type of PAP therapy, pulmonary function, baseline Pa_{CO_2} and Pa_{O_2}, and adherence to therapy.[56]

A recent study tried to identify patient factors that predicted a better response to NIPPV as opposed to CPAP. After evaluating 24 OHS patients, investigators could identify subtypes most likely to respond to CPAP and NIPPV. Patients responding to CPAP have better spirometry and a higher AHI than those who didn't respond. Meanwhile, patients who responded to NIPPV had a higher degree of nocturnal desaturation.[88]

Other modes of NIPPV have recently been investigated in patients with OHS, and may be an alternative for nonresponders to traditional NIPPV. The use of the average volume-assured pressure support (AVAPS) mode allows for consistent tidal volume delivery and has been shown to decrease ventilatory workload as measured by the pressure-time product, mechanical work per liter of ventilation, and work per minute in intubated patients with acute respiratory failure.[89] This mode of NIPPV was studied in patients with OHS who had failed to respond to CPAP therapy as defined by failure to improve $Paco_2$ to less than 45 mm Hg and failure to reduce the respiratory disturbance index to less than 10. Ten patients were randomly assigned to two types of nocturnal ventilation in the spontaneous-timed (S/T) mode (bi-level PAP–S/T) with and without AVAPS in a crossover design for 6 weeks on each mode. AVAPS was set to maintain a tidal volume of 7 to 10 mL/kg and EPAP and respiratory frequency settings were unchanged. In comparison to CPAP therapy, the use of bi-level PAP–S/T resulted in significant increases in slow-wave sleep and REM sleep. In comparison to baseline, mean transcutaneous and daytime $Paco_2$ values did not change significantly with bi-level PAP–S/T but did improve with bi-level PAP–S/T with AVAPS.[90]

Long-Term Management

As outlined above, most patients initially presenting with OHS can be treated with CPAP. For those also with acute respiratory failure or chronic respiratory failure with hypoxemia despite CPAP, the use of bi-level PAP is advocated. Perez de Llano[80] found that at the follow-up visit (at 50 months, range 12–105 months) many patients initially treated with NIPPV for acute decompensation could be maintained on CPAP. Other studies have found that within 7 to 18 days, many patients treated with NIPPV could be maintained on CPAP therapy. After stabilization, follow-up of these patients is recommended for monitoring improvement in their clinical symptoms, arterial blood gases, and serum bicarbonate.[56] Because of the variability in tolerance and response to NIPPV, other means of therapy may need to be considered in place of or in conjunction with NIPPV.

Weight Management and Bariatric Surgery

Obesity remains the central derangement in the pathogenesis of obstructive sleep-disordered breathing and attempts at weight loss should be advocated for all patients with OHS. This has been shown to be an effective therapy for both OSA and for OHS. In a subset of the Wisconsin Sleep Cohort followed over 4 years, a 10% gain in weight resulted in a 32% increase in AHI, while a 10% reduction in weight resulted in a 26% reduction in AHI, regardless of the baseline AHI.[91] The mechanism behind the beneficial effects of weight loss involve reduced airway collapsibility by decreasing the critical airway closing pressure.[92] Dietary weight reduction has been shown to be an effective method of weight loss resulting in improvements in AHI, nocturnal desaturations, and hypercapnia.[93–95] However, long-term maintenance of weight loss has been less effective. In most studies, only a small percentage of patients were able to maintain dietary weight reduction.[96] Interestingly, some patients who maintained their weight loss developed a recurrence of their OSA as manifested by an increase in their AHI.[96] Surgical approaches to weight loss have been shown to be more effective in terms of degree of weight loss and in longer term maintenance of weight loss. A significant number of patients undergoing bariatric surgery have OSA and OHS.[97,98] Bariatric surgery in these patients has also been shown to be effective in reducing the AHI, improving pulmonary function, improving arterial Pao_2 and $Paco_2$ as well as reducing secondary polycythemia.[97] In addition, weight loss after bariatric surgery resulted in improvements in pulmonary hypertension with a significant reduction in mean pulmonary artery pressure and pulmonary arterial occlusion pressure.[99] Improvements in Epworth Sleepiness Scale score were seen as early as 1 month postoperatively.[100] In a long-term study of 38 OHS patients followed on average for 5.8 years after bariatric surgery, 29 were asymptomatic and demonstrated significant improvements in AHI, Pao_2, and $Paco_2$ that were maintained at the end of the study.[28] In a recent meta-analysis of the effects of bariatric surgery, the percentage of patients in the total population whose OSA resolved or improved was 83.6% (95% CI, 71.8%–95.4%).[101] A study of patients with OSA followed for 7.5 years after surgery (range 5–10 years), found that some patients, despite a maintained weight loss after surgery, developed a significantly increased AHI.[102]

The net effect of the multiple comorbid conditions present in many patients with OHS patients is to increase the risk of perioperative complications and increase length of hospital stay.[103,104] Patients with OHS have been shown to have a higher operative mortality than did patients without pulmonary dysfunction (2.4% vs. 0.2% after gastric bypass).[28] In addition, sleep apnea and obesity hypoventilation were both shown to be risk factors for mortality after gastric bypass surgery.[105] A recently validated scoring system for perioperative risk in patients undergoing bariatric surgery includes obesity hypoventilation as a risk factor based on its relationship to the increased incidence of pulmonary embolism.[106] Analysis of prospective data on 3861 patients undergoing bariatric procedures between 1980 and 2004 found that pulmonary embolism–related mortality was 27% and univariate analysis showed that OHS, anastomotic leak, and chronic venous insufficiency were associated with an increased risk of pulmonary embolism.[107,108] The use of CPAP in the perioperative period has not been shown to increase complications in patients undergoing bariatric surgery.[109] As a result, many advocate the routine use of PAP or NIPPV in the preoperative period, immediately after extubation, and in the postoperative period to minimize the risk of perioperative respiratory failure.

Tracheostomy and Airway Surgery

Other surgical approaches to OSA have been tried in patients with OHS. In a study of eight patients with OSA and chronic hypercapnia, seven patients received tracheotomy and one received CPAP therapy.[27] After 6 months, the patients were reevaluated. All patients had improvement in hypersomnolence, snoring, and edema. Polysomnography showed improved REM and slow-wave sleep. Four patients had improvement in their hypercapnia and normalization of serum bicarbonate within 2 weeks of initiating therapy that persisted for 28 to 60 months. However the other four patients remained hypercapnic through their follow-up period of 16 to 48 months. There were no differences between the groups in terms of apnea index before therapy, apnea index after therapy, lowest oxygen desaturation, pulmonary function, changes in dead space due to the tracheotomy tube, or changes in ventilatory responses to carbon dioxide. The patients who failed to show improvement had reduced awake ventilation in comparison to those who responded to therapy.

A retrospective study evaluated the effects of tracheostomy in patients with severe uncomplicated OSA as well as in patients with complicated OSA, defined by the presence of daytime hypoxemia, hypercapnia, or heart failure. Tracheostomy was effective in eliminating significant sleep apnea (AHI < 20) in the patients with uncomplicated OSA. In the OHS patients, the AHI, although improved from baseline and in comparison with having the tracheostomy tube capped, remained elevated (>20) in half of the patients. In addition, although pH and $Paco_2$ levels were improved, the Pao_2 remained unchanged. This ongoing sleep-disordered breathing was thought to be related to periods of hypoventilation.[110] The effects of airway reconstructive surgeries were reported in a retrospective review of 21 morbidly obese patients undergoing a two-phase airway reconstructive surgery involving maxillomandibular advancement and genioglossal advancement.[111] Seventeen

patients (81%) did not require further therapy, 2 patients were maintained on CPAP, and 2 patients, reported to have OHS, were noted to be treatment failures with a persistently elevated AHI and ongoing nocturnal desaturation. Given these results, and the effectiveness of NIPPV, surgical therapy for OHS remains limited and patients undergoing tracheostomy require follow-up monitoring for ongoing uncorrected sleep-disordered breathing related to hypoventilation.

Medical Therapy

The effects of medical therapies in patients with OHS are poorly studied. Medroxyprogesterone (MPA) is thought to have respiratory stimulant properties that may also affect airway muscle tone. It has been shown to increase the ventilatory response to hypoxemia and hypercapnia in normal men.[112] Several small studies have shown that MPA improved oxygenation and hypercapnia in patients with OHS.[113,114] Four of nine patients with OSA showed improvement in apneas with MPA. Three of the patients showing improvement had hypercapnia.[115] Later studies showed no effects on apnea in normocapnic patients and in hypercapnic patients.[116,117] Three OHS patients who did not respond to tracheostomy of CPAP were treated with MPA but did not show improvement in $Paco_2$, response to carbon dioxide rebreathing, or awake minute ventilation.[27] The potential beneficial effects must be weighed against potential side effects, including thromboembolic disease.

The carbonic anhydrase inhibitor acetazolamide has not been well studied in OHS patients. The mechanism of action is thought be stimulation of the ventilatory response via induction of a metabolic acidosis. It may also shift the hypercapnic ventilatory response to a lower carbon dioxide level. It did show normalization of hypercapnia in 1 patient previously nonresponsive to tracheostomy or CPAP.[27] Other studies have shown mixed results in response to hypercapnia and hypoxemia with improvement in central apneas and obstructive apneas.[118,119] Theophylline is thought to act as a respiratory stimulant and may also have positive effects on respiratory muscle function. In 1150 patients with OSA, theophylline was shown to initially reduce AHI, but over a follow-up period of 3 and 28 months, the number of apneas increased slightly on average. Patients with an apnea index of less than 20 had the most benefit.[120] In comparison to CPAP, theophylline showed improvement but not normalization of AHI and desaturation index and CPAP was more effective than theophylline in treating all respiratory variables and in normalizing sleep maintenance and sleep architecture in OSA. Studies in OHS are lacking.[121]

SUMMARY

Given the increasing prevalence of obesity, the numbers of patients with obesity hypoventilation can also be expected to increase. Although advances in understanding the pathophysiology of OHS have been made, the mechanisms behind OHS remain only partly understood. As this condition is associated with significant morbidity and mortality, considering the diagnosis of OHS during the evaluation of patients with obesity and sleep-disordered breathing is essential. Instituting early, appropriate therapy with PAP as well as long-term weight-management strategies can have a significant positive impact on quality of life and patient outcomes.

REFERENCES

1. Formiguera X, Canton A. Obesity: epidemiology and clinical aspects. Best Pract Res Clin Gastroenterol 2004;18(6):1125–46.
2. Flegal KM, Carroll MD, Ogden CL, et al. Prevalence and trends in obesity among US adults. JAMA 2002;288(14):1723–7.
3. Cuvelier A, Muir JF. Acute and chronic respiratory failure in patients with obesity-hypoventilation syndrome: a new challenge for noninvasive ventilation. Chest 2005;128(2):483–5.
4. Solomon CG, Manson JE. Obesity and mortality: a review of the epidemiologic data. Am J Clin Nutr 1997;66(Suppl 4):1044S–50S.
5. Calle EE, Thun MJ, Petrelli JM, et al. Body-mass index and mortality in a prospective cohort of U.S. adults. N Engl J Med 1999;341(15):1097–105.
6. Bickelmann AG, Burwell CS, Robin ED, et al. Extreme obesity associated with alveolar hypoventilation; a Pickwickian syndrome. Am J Med 1956;21(5):811–8.
7. Lavie P. Who was the first to use the term Pickwickian in connection with sleepy patients? History of sleep apnoea syndrome. Sleep Med Rev 2008;12(1):5–17.
8. MacGregor MI, Block AJ, Ball WC Jr. Topics in clinical medicine: serious complications and sudden death in the Pickwickian syndrome. Johns Hopkins Med J 1970;126(5):279–95.
9. Dickens C. The Posthumous Papers of the Pickwick Club. London, UK: Chapman & Hall; 1837.
10. TAAoS Medicine. International classification of sleep disorders. Diagnostic and coding manual. 2nd edition. Westchester (IL): American Academy of Sleep Medicine; 2005.
11. Sleep-related breathing disorders in adults: recommendations for syndrome definition and measurement techniques in clinical research. The Report of an American Academy of Sleep Medicine Task Force. Sleep 1999;22(5):667–89.
12. Olson AL, Zwillich C. The obesity hypoventilation syndrome. Am J Med 2005;118(9):948–56.
13. Mokhlesi B, Tulaimat A. Recent advances in obesity hypoventilation syndrome. Chest 2007;132(4):1322–36.
14. Mokhlesi B, Tulaimat A, Faibussowitsch I, et al. Obesity hypoventilation syndrome: prevalence and predictors in patients with obstructive sleep apnea. Sleep Breath 2007;11(2):117–24.
15. Nowbar S, Burkart KM, Gonzales R, et al. Obesity-associated hypoventilation in hospitalized patients: prevalence, effects, and outcome. Am J Med 2004;116(1):1–7.
16. Martin TJ, Sanders MH. Chronic alveolar hypoventilation: a review for the clinician. Sleep 1995;18(8):617–34.
17. Hida W, Okabe S, Tatsumi K, et al. Nasal continuous positive airway pressure improves quality of life in obesity hypoventilation syndrome. Sleep Breath 2003;7(1):3–12.
18. Chouri-Pontarollo N, Borel JC, Tamisier R, et al. Impaired objective daytime vigilance in obesity-hypoventilation syndrome: impact of noninvasive ventilation. Chest 2007;131(1):148–55.
19. O'Donnell CP, Schaub CD, Haines AS, et al. Leptin prevents respiratory depression in obesity. Am J Respir Crit Care Med 1999;159(5 Pt 1):1477–84.
20. Miller A, Granada M. In-hospital mortality in the Pickwickian syndrome. Am J Med 1974;56(2):144–50.
21. Berg G, Delaive K, Manfreda J, et al. The use of health-care resources in obesity-hypoventilation syndrome. Chest 2001;120(2):377–83.
22. Perez de Llano LA, Golpe R, Ortiz Piquer M, et al. Short-term and long-term effects of nasal intermittent positive pressure ventilation in patients with obesity-hypoventilation syndrome. Chest 2005;128(2):587–94.
23. Kessler R, Chaouat A, Schinkewitch P, et al. The obesity-hypoventilation syndrome revisited: a prospective study of 34 consecutive cases. Chest 2001;120(2):369–76.
24. Resta O, Foschino-Barbaro MP, Bonfitto P, et al. Prevalence and mechanisms of diurnal hypercapnia in a sample of morbidly obese subjects with obstructive sleep apnoea. Respir Med 2000;94(3):240–6.
25. Teichtahl H. The obesity-hypoventilation syndrome revisited. Chest 2001;120(2):336–9.
26. Budweiser S, Riedl SG, Jorres RA, et al. Mortality and prognostic factors in patients with obesity-hypoventilation syndrome undergoing noninvasive ventilation. J Intern Med 2007;261(4):375–83.

27. Rapoport DM, Garay SM, Epstein H, et al. Hypercapnia in the obstructive sleep apnea syndrome. A reevaluation of the "Pickwickian syndrome". Chest 1986;89(5):627–35.
28. Sugerman HJ, Fairman RP, Sood RK, et al. Long-term effects of gastric surgery for treating respiratory insufficiency of obesity. Am J Clin Nutr 1992; 55(Suppl 2):597S–601.
29. Subramanian S, Strohl KP. A management guideline for obesity-hypoventilation syndromes. Sleep Breath 1999;3(4):131–8.
30. Naimark A, Cherniack RM. Compliance of the respiratory system and its components in health and obesity. J Appl Physiol 1960;15:377–82.
31. Pelosi P, Croci M, Ravagnan I, et al. Total respiratory system, lung, and chest wall mechanics in sedated-paralyzed postoperative morbidly obese patients. Chest 1996;109(1):144–51.
32. Sharp JT, Henry JP, Sweany SK, et al. Effects of mass loading the respiratory system in man. J Appl Physiol 1964;19:959–66.
33. Pelosi P, Croci M, Ravagnan I, et al. Respiratory system mechanics in sedated, paralyzed, morbidly obese patients. J Appl Physiol 1997;82(3): 811–8.
34. Unterborn J. Pulmonary function testing in obesity, pregnancy, and extremes of body habitus. Clin Chest Med 2001;22(4):759–67.
35. Jones RL, Nzekwu MM. The effects of body mass index on lung volumes. Chest 2006;130(3):827–33.
36. Behrakis PK, Baydur A, Jaeger MJ, et al. Lung mechanics in sitting and horizontal body positions. Chest 1983;83(4):643–6.
37. Farebrother MJ, McHardy GJ, Munro JF. Relation between pulmonary gas exchange and closing volume before and after substantial weight loss in obese subjects. Br Med J 1974;3(5927):391–3.
38. Saydain G, Beck KC, Decker PA, et al. Clinical significance of elevated diffusing capacity. Chest 2004; vol. 125:446–52.
39. Rubinstein I, Zamel N, DuBarry L, et al. Airflow limitation in morbidly obese, nonsmoking men. Ann Intern Med 1990;112(11):828.
40. Schwartz AR, Patil SP, Laffan AM, et al. Obesity and obstructive sleep apnea: pathogenic mechanisms and therapeutic approaches. Proc Am Thorac Soc 2008;5(2):185–92.
41. Sharp JT, Henry JP, Sweany SK, et al. The total work of breathing in normal and obese men. J Clin Invest 1964;43:728–39.
42. Burki NK, Baker RW. Ventilatory regulation in eucapnic morbid obesity. Am Rev Respir Dis 1984; 129(4):538–43.
43. Chapman KR, Himal HS, Rebuck AS. Ventilatory responses to hypercapnia and hypoxia in patients with eucapnic morbid obesity before and after weight loss. Clin Sci Lond 1990;78(6):541–5.
44. Zwillich CW, Sutton FD, Pierson DJ, et al. Decreased hypoxic ventilatory drive in the obesity-hypoventilation syndrome. Am J Med 1975;59(3):343–8.
45. Akashiba T, Kawahara S, Kosaka N, et al. Determinants of chronic hypercapnia in Japanese men with obstructive sleep apnea syndrome. Chest 2002; 121(2):415–21.
46. Javaheri S, Colangelo G, Lacey W, et al. Chronic hypercapnia in obstructive sleep apnea-hypopnea syndrome. Sleep 1994;17(5):416–23.
47. Marti-Valeri C, Sabate A, Masdevall C, et al. Improvement of associated respiratory problems in morbidly obese patients after open Roux-en-Y gastric bypass. Obes Surg 2007;17(8):1102–10.
48. Heinemann F, Budweiser S, Dobroschke J, et al. Non-invasive positive pressure ventilation improves lung volumes in the obesity hypoventilation syndrome. Respir Med 2007;101(6):1229–35.
49. Sin DD, Jones RL, Man GC. Hypercapnic ventilatory response in patients with and without obstructive sleep apnea: Do age, gender, obesity, and daytime PaCO(2) matter? Chest 2000;117(2):454–9.
50. Krieger J, Sforza E, Apprill M, et al. Pulmonary hypertension, hypoxemia, and hypercapnia in obstructive sleep apnea patients. Chest 1989;96(4): 729–37.
51. Kawata N, Tatsumi K, Terada J, et al. Daytime hypercapnia in obstructive sleep apnea syndrome. Chest 2007;132(6):1832–8.
52. Bradley TD, Rutherford R, Lue F, et al. Role of diffuse airway obstruction in the hypercapnia of obstructive sleep apnea. Am Rev Respir Dis 1986; 134(5):920–4.
53. Berger KI, Ayappa I, Sorkin IB, et al. CO(2) homeostasis during periodic breathing in obstructive sleep apnea. J Appl Physiol 2000;88(1):257–64.
54. Berger KI, Norman RG, Ayappa I, et al. Potential mechanism for transition between acute hypercapnia during sleep to chronic hypercapnia during wakefulness in obstructive sleep apnea. Adv Exp Med Biol 2008;605:431–6.
55. Piper AJ, Wang D, Yee BJ, et al. Randomised trial of CPAP vs bilevel support in the treatment of obesity hypoventilation syndrome without severe nocturnal desaturation. Thorax 2008.
56. Mokhlesi B, Tulaimat A, Evans AT, et al. Impact of adherence with positive airway pressure therapy on hypercapnia in obstructive sleep apnea. J Clin Sleep Med 2006;2(1):57–62.
57. Han F, Chen E, Wei H, et al. Treatment effects on carbon dioxide retention in patients with obstructive sleep apnea-hypopnea syndrome. Chest 2001;119(6):1814–9.
58. Redolfi S, Corda L, La Piana G, et al. Long-term non-invasive ventilation increases chemosensitivity and leptin in obesity-hypoventilation syndrome. Respir Med 2007;101(6):1191–5.

59. Spicuzza L, Bernardi L, Balsamo R, et al. Effect of treatment with nasal continuous positive airway pressure on ventilatory response to hypoxia and hypercapnia in patients with sleep apnea syndrome. Chest 2006;130(3):774–9.

60. Zhang Y, Proenca R, Maffei M, et al. Positional cloning of the mouse obese gene and its human homologue. Nature 1994;372(6505):425–32.

61. Campfield LA, Smith FJ, Guisez Y, et al. Recombinant mouse OB protein: evidence for a peripheral signal linking adiposity and central neural networks. Science 1995;269(5223):546–9.

62. Halaas JL, Gajiwala KS, Maffei M, et al. Weight-reducing effects of the plasma protein encoded by the obese gene. Science 1995;269(5223): 543–6.

63. Tankersley C, Kleeberger S, Russ B, et al. Modified control of breathing in genetically obese (ob/ob) mice. J Appl Physiol 1996;81(2):716–23.

64. Tankersley CG, O'Donnell C, Daood MJ, et al. Leptin attenuates respiratory complications associated with the obese phenotype. J Appl Physiol 1998; 85(6):2261–9.

65. Montague CT, Farooqi IS, Whitehead JP, et al. Congenital leptin deficiency is associated with severe early-onset obesity in humans. Nature 1997; 387(6636):903–8.

66. Clement K, Vaisse C, Lahlou N, et al. A mutation in the human leptin receptor gene causes obesity and pituitary dysfunction. Nature 1998;392(6674): 398–401.

67. Frederich RC, Lollmann B, Hamann A, et al. Expression of ob mRNA and its encoded protein in rodents. Impact of nutrition and obesity. J Clin Invest 1995;96(3):1658–63.

68. Considine RV, Sinha MK, Heiman ML, et al. Serum immunoreactive-leptin concentrations in normal-weight and obese humans. N Engl J Med 1996; 334(5):292–5.

69. Monti V, Carlson JJ, Hunt SC, et al. Relationship of ghrelin and leptin hormones with body mass index and waist circumference in a random sample of adults. J Am Diet Assoc 2006;106(6):822–8.

70. Phipps PR, Starritt E, Caterson I, et al. Association of serum leptin with hypoventilation in human obesity. Thorax 2002;57(1):75–6.

71. Shimura R, Tatsumi K, Nakamura A, et al. Fat accumulation, leptin, and hypercapnia in obstructive sleep apnea-hypopnea syndrome. Chest 2005; 127(2):543–9.

72. Campo A, Fruhbeck G, Zulueta JJ, et al. Hyperleptinaemia, respiratory drive and hypercapnic response in obese patients. Eur Respir J 2007; 30(2):223–31.

73. Banks WA, DiPalma CR, Farrell CL. Impaired transport of leptin across the blood-brain barrier in obesity. Peptides 1999;20(11):1341–5.

74. Caro JF, Kolaczynski JW, Nyce MR, et al. Decreased cerebrospinal-fluid/serum leptin ratio in obesity: a possible mechanism for leptin resistance. Lancet 1996;348(9021):159–61.

75. Schwartz MW, Peskind E, Raskind M, et al. Cerebrospinal fluid leptin levels: relationship to plasma levels and to adiposity in humans. Nat Med 1996; 2(5):589–93.

76. Frederich RC, Hamann A, Anderson S, et al. Leptin levels reflect body lipid content in mice: evidence for diet-induced resistance to leptin action. Nat Med 1995;1(12):1311–4.

77. Yee BJ, Cheung J, Phipps P, et al. Treatment of obesity hypoventilation syndrome and serum leptin. Respiration 2006;73(2):209–12.

78. Berger KI, Ayappa I, Chatr-Amontri B, et al. Obesity hypoventilation syndrome as a spectrum of respiratory disturbances during sleep. Chest 2001;120(4): 1231–8.

79. Waldhorn RE. Nocturnal nasal intermittent positive pressure ventilation with bi-level positive airway pressure (BiPAP) in respiratory failure. Chest 1992;101(2):516–21.

80. Piper AJ, Sullivan CE. Effects of short-term NIPPV in the treatment of patients with severe obstructive sleep apnea and hypercapnia. Chest 1994;105(2): 434–40.

81. Schafer H, Ewig S, Hasper E, et al. Failure of CPAP therapy in obstructive sleep apnoea syndrome: predictive factors and treatment with bilevel-positive airway pressure. Respir Med 1998;92(2): 208–15.

82. Sullivan CE, Berthon-Jones M, Issa FG. Remission of severe obesity-hypoventilation syndrome after short-term treatment during sleep with nasal continuous positive airway pressure. Am Rev Respir Dis 1983;128(1):177–81.

83. Shivaram U, Cash ME, Beal A. Nasal continuous positive airway pressure in decompensated hypercapnic respiratory failure as a complication of sleep apnea. Chest 1993;104(3):770–4.

84. Masa JF, Celli BR, Riesco JA, et al. The obesity hypoventilation syndrome can be treated with noninvasive mechanical ventilation. Chest 2001;119(4): 1102–7.

85. Masa JF, Celli BR, Riesco JA, et al. Noninvasive positive pressure ventilation and not oxygen may prevent overt ventilatory failure in patients with chest wall diseases. Chest 1997;112(1): 207–13.

86. Banerjee D, Yee BJ, Piper AJ, et al. Obesity hypoventilation syndrome: hypoxemia during continuous positive airway pressure. Chest 2007; 131(6):1678–84.

87. Guo YF, Sforza E, Janssens JP. Respiratory patterns during sleep in obesity-hypoventilation patients treated with nocturnal pressure

support: a preliminary report. Chest 2007; 131(4):1090–9.

88. Perez de Llano LA, Golpe R, Piquer MO, et al. Clinical heterogeneity among patients with obesity hypoventilation syndrome: therapeutic implications. Respiration 2008;75(1):34–9.

89. Amato MB, Barbas CS, Bonassa J, et al. Volume-assured pressure support ventilation (VAPSV). A new approach for reducing muscle workload during acute respiratory failure. Chest 1992;102(4): 1225–34.

90. Storre JH, Seuthe B, Fiechter R, et al. Average volume-assured pressure support in obesity hypoventilation: a randomized crossover trial. Chest 2006; 130(3):815–21.

91. Peppard PE, Young T, Palta M, et al. Longitudinal study of moderate weight change and sleep-disordered breathing. JAMA 2000;284(23): 3015–21.

92. Schwartz AR, Gold AR, Schubert N, et al. Effect of weight loss on upper airway collapsibility in obstructive sleep apnea. Am Rev Respir Dis 1991; 144(3 Pt 1):494–8.

93. Smith PL, Gold AR, Meyers DA, et al. Weight loss in mildly to moderately obese patients with obstructive sleep apnea. Ann Intern Med 1985;103(6 Pt 1): 850–5.

94. Kansanen M, Vanninen E, Tuunainen A, et al. The effect of a very low-calorie diet-induced weight loss on the severity of obstructive sleep apnoea and autonomic nervous function in obese patients with obstructive sleep apnoea syndrome. Clin Physiol 1998;18(4):377–85.

95. Harman EM, Wynne JW, Block AJ. The effect of weight loss on sleep-disordered breathing and oxygen desaturation in morbidly obese men. Chest 1982;82(3):291–4.

96. Sampol G, Munoz X, Sagales MT, et al. Long-term efficacy of dietary weight loss in sleep apnoea/hypopnoea syndrome. Eur Respir J 1998;12(5):1156–9.

97. Sugerman HJ, Fairman RP, Baron PL, et al. Gastric surgery for respiratory insufficiency of obesity. Chest 1986;90(1):81–6.

98. Frey WC, Pilcher J. Obstructive sleep-related breathing disorders in patients evaluated for bariatric surgery. Obes Surg 2003;13(5):676–83.

99. Sugerman HJ, Baron PL, Fairman RP, et al. Hemodynamic dysfunction in obesity hypoventilation syndrome and the effects of treatment with surgically induced weight loss. Ann Surg 1988;207(5): 604–13.

100. Varela JE, Hinojosa MW, Nguyen NT. Resolution of obstructive sleep apnea after laparoscopic gastric bypass. Obes Surg 2007;17(10):1279–82.

101. Buchwald H, Avidor Y, Braunwald E, et al. Bariatric surgery: a systematic review and meta-analysis. JAMA 2004;292(14):1724–37.

102. Pillar G, Peled R, Lavie P. Recurrence of sleep apnea without concomitant weight increase 7.5 years after weight reduction surgery. Chest 1994;106(6): 1702–4.

103. Cawley J, Sweeney MJ, Kurian M, et al. Predicting complications after bariatric surgery using obesity-related co-morbidities. Obes Surg 2007;17(11): 1451–6.

104. Ballantyne GH, Svahn J, Capella RF, et al. Predictors of prolonged hospital stay following open and laparoscopic gastric bypass for morbid obesity: body mass index, length of surgery, sleep apnea, asthma, and the metabolic syndrome. Obes Surg 2004;14(8):1042–50.

105. DeMaria EJ, Portenier D, Wolfe L. Obesity surgery mortality risk score: proposal for a clinically useful score to predict mortality risk in patients undergoing gastric bypass. Surg Obes Relat Dis 2007; 3(2):134–40.

106. DeMaria EJ, Murr M, Byrne TK, et al. Validation of the obesity surgery mortality risk score in a multicenter study proves it stratifies mortality risk in patients undergoing gastric bypass for morbid obesity. Ann Surg 2007;246(4):578–82 [discussion: 583–4].

107. Carmody BJ, Sugerman HJ, Kellum JM, et al. Pulmonary embolism complicating bariatric surgery: detailed analysis of a single institution's 24-year experience. J Am Coll Surg 2006; 203(6):831–7.

108. Sapala JA, Wood MH, Schuhknecht MP, et al. Fatal pulmonary embolism after bariatric operations for morbid obesity: a 24-year retrospective analysis. Obes Surg 2003;13(6):819–25.

109. Huerta S, DeShields S, Shpiner R, et al. Safety and efficacy of postoperative continuous positive airway pressure to prevent pulmonary complications after Roux-en-Y gastric bypass. J Gastrointest Surg 2002;6(3):354–8.

110. Kim SH, Eisele DW, Smith PL, et al. Evaluation of patients with sleep apnea after tracheotomy. Arch Otolaryngol Head Neck Surg 1998;124(9): 996–1000.

111. Li KK, Powell NB, Riley RW, et al. Morbidly obese patients with severe obstructive sleep apnea: is airway reconstructive surgery a viable treatment option? Laryngoscope 2000;110(6):982–7.

112. Zwillich CW, Natalino MR, Sutton FD, et al. Effects of progesterone on chemosensitivity in normal men. J Lab Clin Med 1978;92(2):262–9.

113. Lyons HA, Huang CT. Therapeutic use of progesterone in alveolar hypoventilation associated with obesity. Am J Med 1968;44(6):881–8.

114. Sutton FD Jr, Zwillich CW, Creagh CE, et al. Progesterone for outpatient treatment of Pickwickian syndrome. Ann Intern Med 1975;83(4): 476–9.

115. Strohl KP, Hensley MJ, Saunders NA, et al. Progesterone administration and progressive sleep apneas. JAMA 1981;245(12):1230–2.

116. Rajagopal KR, Abbrecht PH, Jabbari B. Effects of medroxyprogesterone acetate in obstructive sleep apnea. Chest 1986;90(6):815–21.

117. Cook WR, Benich JJ, Wooten SA. Indices of severity of obstructive sleep apnea syndrome do not change during medroxyprogesterone acetate therapy. Chest 1989;96(2):262–6.

118. Tojima H, Kunitomo F, Kimura H, et al. Effects of acetazolamide in patients with the sleep apnoea syndrome. Thorax 1988;43(2):113–9.

119. Whyte KF, Gould GA, Airlie MA, et al. Role of protriptyline and acetazolamide in the sleep apnea/hypopnea syndrome. Sleep 1988;11(5):463–72.

120. Meissner P, Dorow P, Thalhofer S, et al. [Theophylline acceptance in long-term therapy of patients with obstructive sleep related respiratory disorder]. Pneumologie 1995;49(Suppl 1):187–9 [in German].

121. Saletu B, Oberndorfer S, Anderer P, et al. Efficiency of continuous positive airway pressure versus theophylline therapy in sleep apnea: comparative sleep laboratory studies on objective and subjective sleep and awakening quality. Neuropsychobiology 1999;39(3):151–9.

Sleep in Patients with Respiratory Muscle Weakness

Himanshu Desai, MD[a], M. Jeffery Mador, MD[b],*

KEYWORDS

- Respiratory muscle weakness • Neuromuscular disorders
- Sleep-disordered breathing
- Sleep related alveolar hypoventilation • Polysomnogram
- Noninvasive positive pressure ventilation
- Amyotrophic lateral sclerosis
- Myasthenia gravis • Duchenne's muscular dystrophy
- Myotonic dystrophy • Phrenic nerve palsy
- Post-polio syndrome

Patients with respiratory muscle weakness are at high risk of developing hypoxemia and hypercapnia during sleep. Most of these patients remain undiagnosed and untreated despite the high incidence of sleep related breathing disorders. Sleep-disordered breathing (SDB) is a significant cause of morbidity and mortality in these patients.[1–4] SDB is most often due to nocturnal hypoventilation. However, nocturnal hypoventilation may be complicated by obstructive sleep apnea (OSA) or central sleep apnea (CSA).[5–7] In some patients, sleep apnea per se may be the predominant abnormality. All humans are vulnerable to respiratory impairment in sleep, particularly rapid-eye-movement (REM) sleep.[8] Patients with respiratory muscle weakness are particularly at risk as they are predisposed to serious perturbations of homeostasis during sleep.[9–12] Sleep-related physiologic changes interact with a compromised neuromuscular system to create conditions that result in different forms of sleep-related hypoxemia and sleep fragmentation. In more severe cases, patients may also have alveolar hypoventilation while awake, which can lead to progressive hypercapnia and ultimately, to respiratory failure.[13] Despite the high incidence of SDB in this population group, most patients are not appropriately diagnosed.[14] It is important to recognize these problems at an early stage because they are correctable and because their treatment with relatively simple and noninvasive means can lead to an improved quality of life.[15]

In this chapter, the physiologic effects of sleep on respiratory muscle activity and breathing are described. The evidence of disruption of sleep architecture, SDB and nocturnal oxygenation in patients with respiratory muscle weakness is reviewed. Finally, the more specific findings in various diseases, and the evaluation and management of these conditions, are described.

EFFECTS OF SLEEP ON RESPIRATORY MUSCLES AND BREATHING

Control of respiration during sleep and wakefulness depends on two anatomically and functionally independent systems: the metabolic (automatic) and behavioral (voluntary) systems.[16] Both systems are active during wakefulness,

[a] Division of Pulmonary, Critical Care and Sleep Medicine, Department of Medicine, State University of New York at Buffalo, 3495 Bailey Avenue, Buffalo, NY 14215, USA
[b] Division of Pulmonary, Critical Care and Sleep Medicine, Department of Medicine, Veterans Affairs Western New York Health Care System and University at Buffalo, State University of New York, 3495 Bailey Avenue, Buffalo, NY 14215, USA
* Corresponding author.
E-mail address: mador@buffalo.edu (M.J. Mador).

Sleep Med Clin 3 (2008) 541–550
doi:10.1016/j.jsmc.2008.08.010
1556-407X/08/$ – see front matter. Published by Elsevier Inc.

whereas the metabolic system predominates during sleep. Respiratory homeostasis is vulnerable to minor changes that can occur during sleep.

Non-Rapid Eye Movement Sleep

At sleep onset, phasic diaphragmatic, intercostals, and genioglossus activity fall and then rise again, while phasic and tonic activity of tensor palatini (an upper airway dilator muscle) falls abruptly and remains low.[17] Decreased activity of the tensor palatini muscle results in increased upper airway resistance. Ventilation falls abruptly and is associated with a more shallow and regular breathing pattern, resulting in a rise in the PCO_2 of an average 2–8 mm Hg.[18,19] Ventilation shows only a slight further decline after sleep becomes established. Upper airway resistance (UAR) increases suddenly at sleep onset because of decreased activity of the upper airway dilator muscles and reduced output from the medullary respiratory neurons to the upper airway muscles during sleep.[20] The increase in phasic diaphragmatic and intercostal EMG activity in non-rapid eye movement (NREM) sleep (following the transient fall at sleep onset) reflects the rise in respiratory workload due to increased UAR. The ventilatory response to hypoxia is decreased during NREM sleep compared with wakefulness in men but not in women.[21,22] There is conflicting evidence regarding ventilatory responsiveness to hypercapnia during NREM sleep. Douglas and colleagues[23] have noted depressed hypercapnic ventilatory responsiveness during NREM sleep in both men and women, although other investigators reported no difference in responsiveness in women during NREM sleep compared with wakefulness.[24]

Rapid Eye Movement Sleep

During rapid eye movement (REM) sleep there is a marked generalized reduction in the tone of skeletal muscles, with the exception of the diaphragm and extra-ocular muscles.[25] Thus, during REM sleep, the principal burden for maintaining ventilation is on the diaphragm. REM sleep comprises phasic REM associated with bursts of rapid eye movements, and tonic REM, between bursts of rapid eye movements. In comparison to tonic REM, phasic REM is associated with smaller tidal volumes, higher respiratory rate, lower minute ventilation, and a more irregular breathing pattern.[26–28] Douglas and colleagues[18] reported a further fall in tidal volume, minute ventilation, and mean inspiratory flow from NREM to REM sleep, while Gould and colleagues[26] and Millman and colleagues[27] reported only a trend for a fall

in tidal volume, with no significant reduction in ventilation during REM compared with NREM sleep. Ventilatory responses to hypercapnia and hypoxia are depressed during REM sleep in both men and women.

The causes of sleep-related alveolar hypoventilation are summarized in **Box 1**. Metabolic rate decreases during sleep but not sufficiently to prevent the increase in pCO2. These sleep-related ventilatory changes do not have clinically important effects in normal individuals. However, they become critical, transforming physiologic nocturnal hypoventilation into pathologic sleep-related hypoventilation, abnormal breathing patterns, and respiratory failure in patients with respiratory muscle weakness.

CAUSES OF RESPIRATORY MUSCLE WEAKNESS

The respiratory muscles consist principally of the diaphragm, the intercostal, abdominal, and accessory muscles. They differ from other skeletal muscles in that they contract throughout life, rhythmically driving the chest wall without—in the case of the diaphragm—any periods of rest.[29] Respiratory muscle weakness can be caused by lesions at any level in the pathway connecting the respiratory centers to the respiratory muscles. Respiratory muscle dysfunction may occur as a result of cerebral or cerebellar lesions.[30,31] Central nervous system disorders that can cause respiratory muscle weakness include: infarction, hemorrhage, demyelination, hypoxia, and external compression. Peripheral nervous system disorders that can cause respiratory muscle weakness are outlined in **Table 1**.

SLEEP IN PATIENTS WITH RESPIRATORY MUSCLE WEAKNESS

Patients with respiratory muscle weakness have reduced total sleep time and sleep efficiency.[32,33] Marked sleep fragmentation with frequent arousals is commonly seen in patients with respiratory or sleep-related symptoms.[32–34] Complete suppression of REM sleep has been reported in association with severe diaphragmatic weakness.[35,36] This may represent a compensatory

---

Box 1
Causes of sleep related alveolar hypoventilation

- Loss of wakefulness stimuli
- Increased upper airway resistance
- Impaired chemo responsiveness of the respiratory neurons

Table 1
Peripheral nervous system disorders causing respiratory muscle weakness

Site of Lesion	Diseases
Spinal cord	Trauma, Tumor, Syringomyelia, Multiple sclerosis, Poliomyelitis, Amyotrophic lateral sclerosis, Tetanus
Motor nerves	Phrenic nerve injury (trauma, surgery, tumor), Gullain-Barre syndrome, Diphtheria, Nutritional polyneuropathies (beriberi), Carcinomatous neuropathy, Critical illness polyneuropathy, Lyme disease
Neuromuscular junction	Myasthenia gravis, Lambert-Eaton syndrome, Botulism, Tick paralysis, Organophosphate poisoning
Muscles	Congenital myopathies (acid-maltase deficiency, mitochondrial myopathy), Myotonic dystrophy, Muscular dystrophies, Polymyositis/Dermatomyositis, Other collagen vascular diseases, Malnutrition, Endocrine diseases (hypo-hyper thyroidism, exogenous steroids, Addison's disease, etc.), Electrolytes abnormalities (calcium, phosphate or magnesium depletion)

mechanism because these subjects are most vulnerable to oxygen desaturation during REM sleep. Patients with respiratory muscle weakness also have abnormally low lung and chest wall compliance.[37–39] Reduced lung compliance has been attributed to microatelectasis and focal pulmonary parenchymal fibrosis. Reduced chest wall compliance may be related to increased stiffness of the rib cage. These changes lead to increased work of breathing at any given level of minute ventilation.

A high prevalence of SDB has been reported in neuromuscular diseases, irrespective of the primary disorder.[5,14,32–34,40,41] The most common SDB in patients with respiratory muscle weakness is sleep-related, especially REM –related, hypoventilation.[10,33] Both central and obstructive apneas can also occur.[5,33,34,36,41]

The effects of normal sleep-related physiologic changes are accentuated in patients with respiratory muscle weakness. While patients are awake, both voluntary and metabolic respiratory controls are intact; and the central respiratory neurons increase their rate of firing or recruit additional respiratory neurons to sufficiently drive weak respiratory muscles to adequately maintain ventilation.[42] However, during sleep, respiration is dependent primarily on the metabolic control system, as voluntary control is depressed, making the system more vulnerable and potentially leading to severe hypoventilation and the development of apnea-hypopneas.[8]

Central hypopneas are the most frequently reported sleep-breathing event in patients with respiratory muscle weakness, which are more frequent and prolonged in REM sleep.[5,33,41,43,44] Relative hypotonia of the intercostals and accessory respiratory muscles combined with insufficient diaphragmatic recruitment leads to

hypoventilation during REM sleep. The degree of muscle suppression during REM sleep, and consequent reduction in ventilation, is proportional to the density of eye movements.[26,27] The degree of desaturation is related to the severity of diaphragmatic weakness.[9,36] An increase in upper airway resistance and obstructive sleep apnea may develop as a result of weakness of pharyngeal muscle dilators, resulting in a tendency of the pharyngeal wall to collapse during inspiration. This can be further aggravated by anatomic abnormalities such as tonsillar hypertrophy, obesity, and craniofacial dysmorphisms and micrognathia that reduce the oropharyngeal lumen.[13]

The classification of events as "central" or "obstructive" using noninvasive monitoring is particularly difficult in patients with respiratory muscle weakness. Obstructive apnea may be misclassified as central when respiratory muscles are too weak to move the chest wall against a closed pharynx.[1,41] Severe diaphragmatic weakness causes paradoxical movement of the chest and abdomen even without narrowing of the upper airway, which may cause misclassification of central hypopneas as obstructive. Studies in which esophageal pressure was recorded to accurately determine the nature of events have reported predominantly central events.[5,44]

Potential factors causing sleep-related hypoventilation in respiratory muscle weakness are outlined in **Box 2**.[8]

Specific Findings in Individual Disorders

Post-polio syndrome
Post-polio syndrome refers to new manifestations occurring many years after the acute poliomyelitis infection. It may result in progressive respiratory muscle weakness and bulbar muscle dysfunction.

Box 2
Factors causing sleep-related hypoventilation in respiratory muscle weakness[8]

- Weakness of the respiratory and chest wall muscles causing impaired chest bellows
- Increased work of breathing due to altered chest mechanics
- Hyporesponsive chemoreceptors due to altered afferent inputs from skeletal muscle spindles
- Weakness of upper airway muscles that increases upper airway resistance
- Decrement of minute ventilation and alveolar ventilation during sleep
- REM-related hypotonia and atonia of all the respiratory muscles except for the diaphragm, causing increased diaphragmatic workload
- Respiratory muscle fatigue due to increasing demand on the respiratory muscles during sleep, particularly REM sleep
- Kyphoscoliosis due to neuromuscular disorders causing restrictive ventilatory impairment

Pulmonary problems account for most of the morbidity and mortality.[45,46] Sleep disturbances are common, appearing in 31% of patients, even in those without previous bulbar involvement.[47] Sleep problems in these patients include hypoventilation, apnea, hypopneas, significant oxyhemoglobin desaturation, and excessive daytime sleepiness and sleep disruption.[48] Central sleep apnea has been described in patients who had received ventilatory support during their initial illness as a result of bulbar involvement.[49] However, most apneas are of obstructive or mixed variety with a favorable response to continuous positive airway pressure (CPAP).[12] Sleep studies should be performed in all post-polio patients complaining of sleep disturbance or respiratory manifestations.[12]

Amyotrophic lateral sclerosis

Amyotrophic lateral sclerosis (ALS) is a disease of progressive degeneration of the motor neurons of the spinal cord, brain stem, motor cortex, and corticospinal tracts. ALS is characterized by the presence of both upper and lower motor neuron signs.[50] The reported frequency of sleep disordered breathing is very variable (17%–76%) and appears to reflect the prevalence of respiratory and sleep-related symptoms, and the impairment of daytime respiratory function in the populations studied.[10,32,33,51,52] In the largest unselected cross-sectional study, Gay and colleagues[10] reported a mean Apnea-Hypopnea Index (AHI) of

11.3 per hour in 21 subjects, mostly obstructive or mixed apneas. However, obstructive events were not primarily responsible for nocturnal oxygen desaturation. Hypoventilation was found to be the primary explanation for the decline in oxygen saturation. Diaphragmatic weakness is associated with sleep disruption and a reduction in, or with more extreme weakness, complete suppression of REM sleep.[35] No significant relationships between bulbar involvement and the severity of sleep-disordered breathing or the type of event (obstructive or central) have been reported.[10,32,33,35,51,52] Therefore, nocturnal desaturation and sleep disruption in ALS appear to be due mainly to diaphragmatic weakness and hypoventilation, rather than to bulbar weakness.[35] The SDB in ALS usually will initially respond to bilevel positive airway pressure (bilevel PAP).[32] Of course, ALS is a progressive disease and the patient will eventually develop worsening respiratory failure during the day. In addition, increasing loss of bulbar function is expected. This progression will eventually result in failure of noninvasive ventilation (NIV). If, at that time, the patient elects to continue with aggressive supportive measures, invasive ventilation through a tracheostomy will be required.

Myasthenia gravis

Myasthenia gravis (MG) is an autoimmune disease in which autoantibodies against muscle acetylcholine receptor attack the receptor at the neuromuscular junction resulting in a reduced number of receptors in the postjunctional region. It is characterized by easy fatigability of the muscles due to failure of neuromuscular junction transmission of nerve impulses.[42] Sleep-disordered breathing is common in MG which is associated with peripheral respiratory muscle weakness, particularly diaphragmatic weakness.[1] Patients often have sleep apnea with predominantly mixed and obstructive events, along with oxygen desaturation of moderate severity.[13] Sleep-disordered breathing and nocturnal desaturation are most pronounced during REM sleep,[44,53] when the diaphragm is the only muscle that remains active. Older patients with obesity, lower total lung capacity (TLC) and abnormal daytime arterial blood gases are most vulnerable.[44] Sleep-disordered breathing and nocturnal desaturation may improve following treatment with thymectomy[54] or prednisolone.[53]

The Lambert-Eaton myasthenic syndrome (LEMS) is caused by antibodies to voltage-gated calcium channels on the presynaptic nerve terminal of the motor nerve. SDB has also been described in many patients with LEMS.[8]

Neuropathy and phrenic nerve palsy

Peripheral neuropathies usually present as bilateral, symmetric, with distal sensory signs, and symptoms of muscle weakness and wasting that affect the lower extremities more than the upper extremities.[42] Phrenic nerve damage resulting in diaphragmatic paralysis may be part of the spectrum of involvement in some diffuse neuropathies. Unilateral paralysis is usually asymptomatic unless there is coexisting lung disease. Bilateral paralysis is invariably symptomatic.[13] Patients with isolated diaphragmatic paralysis are particularly prone to nocturnal desaturation during REM sleep,[36] even with only unilateral involvement.[55] As the frequency of oxyhemoglobin desaturation increases during REM sleep, arousals and daytime somnolence become increasingly prominent so that the condition resembles the sleep apnea syndrome. The severity of hypoventilation and the depth of oxygen desaturation during NREM sleep is more pronounced if there are abnormal chest wall mechanics or involvement of the accessory respiratory muscles.[13] Daytime respiratory failure is unusual with isolated bilateral diaphragmatic paralysis unless there is coexisting intrinsic lung disease (eg, COPD) or obesity.[36,55–58]

The diagnosis of bilateral diaphragmatic paralysis is suspected when patients complain of dyspnea that clearly worsens when the patent lies supine and there is no evidence of heart disease. Paradoxical respirations may be seen which are best appreciated in the supine position. There are major discrepancies in vital capacity between the erect and supine postures. In normal subjects, recumbency results in up to a 10% fall in vital capacity compared with the upright value. In contrast, patients with bilateral diaphragmatic paralysis show a 50% decrease in vital capacity in the supine posture. Nocturnal polysomnography is critical for evaluation of the presence and degree of sleep-related respiratory dysfunction in patients with suspected paralysis of the diaphragm.[13] Noninvasive nocturnal positive pressure ventilation usually results in improvement in sleep complaints.

Myotonic dystrophy

Myotonic dystrophy (MD) is an autosomal dominant, multisystem disease affecting skeletal and cardiac muscles as well as CNS structures and endocrine function.[13] Daytime somnolence, hypercapnia, SDB and nocturnal desaturation are all common in MD.[5,59–61] The AHI and degree of nocturnal desaturation are greater than in non-myotonic neuromuscular diseases with a similar degree of respiratory muscle weakness.[60] Patients with MD tend to be heavier than those with other forms of neuromuscular disease,[60] and the degree of nocturnal desaturation is related to the BMI.[59]

Sleep problems in MD are due to both SDB and primary hypersomnia. The SDB has a dual mechanism: weakness and myotonia of respiratory muscles[42] and abnormalities of the central control of ventilation.[62,63] In most patients with MD, sleepiness is not clearly attributable to hypercapnia, SDB, or disturbance of sleep architecture.[60,64] There is evidence to suggest complex, widespread malfunction of the circadian and ultradian timing system[65] including neuroendocrine abnormalities in sleep.[13] Hypersomnia in MD in the absence of untreated sleep disordered breathing may respond successfully to the administration of stimulants such as modafinil or methylphenidate.[66] It is important to evaluate patients with MD with an overnight polysomnogram. A multiple sleep latency test (MSLT) may sometimes be indicated since the excessive daytime sleepiness may not be due solely to SDB.[48]

Duchenne's muscular dystrophy

Duchenne's muscular dystrophy (DMD) is characterized by progressive muscular weakness that ultimately involves all the respiratory muscles leading to substantial morbidity and, eventually, mortality.[67] Patients with DMD also develop restrictive lung disease as muscle weakness progresses and rib cage deformities appear.[13] Patients with DMD suffer from hypoventilation during sleep with hypercapnia and profound oxyhemoglobin desaturation in REM sleep, despite normal awake respiratory function.[7,68] The severity of SDB cannot be predicted from awake pulmonary function tests.[41] Sleep fragmentation, frequent arousals, and REM sleep deprivation also occur in patients with DMD, resulting in excessive daytime sleepiness.[69] Patients with DMD and SDB respond well to noninvasive positive pressure ventilation during sleep.[68]

Nocturnal respiratory dysfunction has been described in patients with other types of muscular dystrophies and primary muscle diseases.

GENERAL DIAGNOSTIC APPROACH
Clinical Evaluation

The initial approach to patients with respiratory muscle weakness with SDB is clinical. The presence of symptoms is the major factor favoring evaluation of the patient for OSA, central sleep apnea or hypoventilation. When clinical features strongly suggest SDB, physical examination must be directed to uncover bulbar and respiratory muscle weakness, including diaphragmatic dysfunction, in addition to a detailed neurologic and general medical examination.[16,70] Nocturnal restlessness, frequent unexplained arousal, loud snoring, excessive daytime sleepiness, prolonged sleep inertia, fatigue, inappropriate napping, and, in the very young, failure to thrive and declining school performance are among these clinical features.[48] However, some patients may have SDB without prominent symptoms but with suggestive physiologic parameters, eg, severe restriction on pulmonary function tests or unexplained cor pulmonale. Patients with a maximal inspiratory pressure (PI max) below 50 percent of predicted, or a forced vital capacity (FVC) below 1–1.5 L due to ALS or other neuromuscular diseases, are more likely to have significant nocturnal desaturation.[10,71–73] Such patients should also be evaluated with an arterial blood gas and a sleep study.

Diagnostic Tests

Arterial blood gas (ABG) analysis, pulmonary function tests, overnight oximetry, portable multichannel devices, and overnight polysomnography in the sleep laboratory are all available, but the optimal test for screening patients with respiratory muscle weakness has not been established.

In the early stages of neuromuscular disorders, ABG values remain normal during wakefulness. Only in the advanced stages with chronic respiratory failure will these values become abnormal.[8] Difference in vital capacity between erect and supine positions during wakefulness and awake ABG values are of limited value in predicting SDB.[48] Overnight oximetry alone may be used to screen for oxygen desaturation associated with nocturnal hypoventilation. Oximetry may underestimate the degree of sleep apnea, however, depending upon the scoring criteria used.[74–77] Portable devices with four or more channels (eg, heart rate, air flow, chest movement, and oximetry) are likely to detect moderate to severe OSA. However, the severity of sleep apnea may be underestimated, and mild disease may be missed entirely. Polysomnography is currently considered the "gold standard" for assessing SDB in patients with neuromuscular symptoms.[9,78,79] In addition to the regular PSG channels, a transcutaneous or end tidal CO_2 channel is very helpful in providing a direct index for hypoventilation.[8,48] Additional EMG channels for the assessment of muscle activity in the accessory respiratory muscles may also be helpful, especially in determining efficacy of treatment. Indications for polysomnography in patients with respiratory muscle weakness are shown in **Box 3**.

> **Box 3**
> **Indications for polysomnography in patients with respiratory muscle weakness**
>
> - Symptoms of sleep disordered breathing
> - $PaCO_2$ >45 mm of Hg on ABG[72,98]
> - Inspiratory vital capacity <40 percent of predicted[72,98]
> - Severely reduced peak inspiratory pressure (PIP <2.5 kPa)[72,98]
> - Unexplained cor pulmonale

Supplemental Tests

In patients with myotonic dystrophy, a multiple sleep latency test may ultimately be required, for evaluating hypersomnolence that is independent of SDB.[48] Phrenic and intercostal nerve conduction studies may detect phrenic or intercostal neuropathy causing respiratory muscle weakness. Needle EMG of the diaphragm may reveal diaphragmatic denervation, suggesting neurogenic dysfunction of the diaphragm.[8] Esophageal pressure monitoring during sleep is helpful in distinguishing central versus obstructive apneas. It is particularly useful in detecting the upper airway resistance syndrome, characterized by subtle increases in respiratory effort that are not manifested by changes in air flow but are associated with arousal and sleep fragmentation.[80]

TREATMENT

The goal of treatment is to eliminate excessive daytime somnolence, improve nocturnal desaturation, improve quality of life, and prevent serious complications of chronic respiratory failure such as pulmonary hypertension and congestive heart failure. In the past, the mainstay of treatment was invasive ventilation through a tracheostomy, but this has been largely replaced by noninvasive positive pressure ventilation (NIPPV). Two types of noninvasive ventilatory support are available: negative and positive pressure ventilation.

Negative Pressure Ventilation

Negative pressure ventilation was first introduced in the 1950s to treat patients with respiratory failure due to acute poliomyelitis. It has been shown to improve oxygenation during NREM sleep. Episodes of severe desaturation still occur during REM sleep, associated with obstructive events. Negative pressure ventilation contributes to upper airway obstruction both in patients with neuromuscular disease[81–83] and in normal individuals[84] because they augment expanding forces to the chest wall but not the upper airway. Negative pressure ventilators are bulky and limit the patient's acceptance. They are also difficult for patients with neuromuscular disease to get in and out of without assistance.

Positive Pressure Ventilation

In uncontrolled studies, positive pressure ventilation has been shown to improve nocturnal saturation, sleep disordered breathing, sleep efficiency, and sleep architecture in neuromuscular disease with respiratory muscle weakness.[85,86] In the Cochrane database of systematic reviews, the authors concluded that mechanical ventilation should be offered as a therapeutic option to patients with chronic hypoventilation due to neuromuscular diseases because the current evidence to support its therapeutic benefit is weak but consistent.[87] The current standard of care for chronic ventilatory failure in patients with respiratory muscle weakness is NIPPV using a nasal mask or prongs.[8] Two types of delivery of positive pressure are available: continuous positive airway pressure (CPAP), and bilevel PAP. CPAP is typically not an effective therapy for nocturnal hypoventilation. Bilevel PAP is a pressure targeted device in which the inspiratory and expiratory pressures can be individually adjusted. The gradient between the inspiratory and expiratory pressures and the compliance of the respiratory system determine the amount by which ventilation is assisted, similar to the pressure support mode on a conventional intensive care ventilator. The start of inspiration is triggered by the patient. A back-up rate can be applied in patients who are at risk of respiratory failure because their spontaneous efforts might become absent or ineffective.

Invasive ventilation using tracheostomy can be considered in patients who are unable to tolerate NIV, unable to clear secretions, or for whom NIV is no longer effective because of progression of their disease.

Daytime ABGs improve with long-term nocturnal ventilation,[85,86,88,89] and are associated with an increased ventilatory response to carbon dioxide.[85] NIV appears to improve survival in patients with hypercarbic respiratory failure due to stable or slowly progressive neuromuscular disease, when compared with historical controls.[90] In more rapidly progressive conditions such as ALS, NIV also appears to prolong survival[91,92] and improve quality of life.[93] Recent consensus guideline suggest that noninvasive positive pressure ventilation should be initiated in patients with clinical symptoms and one of the following

criteria: 1) $PaCO_2 \geq 45$ mm of Hg; 2) nocturnal arterial oxygen saturation ≤ 88 percent for 5 consecutive minutes; and 3) in cases of progressive neuromuscular diseases, maximal inspiratory pressure of <60 cmH_2O or FVC of <50 percent of predicted.[94]

Other Treatment Modalities

The role of supplemental oxygen therapy using low flow oxygen in treatment of SDB in patients with respiratory muscle weakness remains controversial. Supplemental oxygen may improve oxygenation but will not address the underyling cause, which is nocturnal hypoventilation. According to most investigators, oxygen therapy in restrictive thoracic disorders due to neuromuscular diseases is ineffective and may be dangerous, potentially leading to marked CO_2 retention.[95] Supplemental oxygen via nasal cannula may be sufficient in some cases to correct mild REM sleep-related oxygen desaturations.[13]

Patients with myotonic dystrophy may require additional treatment with stimulants for optimal daytime functioning.[66] Modafinil reduces somnolence and improves mood in these patients.[96] For those patients who fail noninvasive positive pressure ventilation or who cannot cooperate with such treatment, tracheostomy may be beneficial. The role of inspiratory muscle training is controversial but in selected patients without rapidly progressive disease, inspiratory muscle training might be useful in the early stages of the disease.[97]

SUMMARY

Patients with respiratory muscle weakness are at high risk for developing SDB, which unfortunately remains under diagnosed. Symptoms related to sleep disruption and hypercapnia are a major cause of morbidity. Polysomnographic evaluation in the sleep laboratory is recommended for symptomatic patients. Most patients with SDB and respiratory muscle weakness respond well to relatively simple and noninvasive methods of treatment, resulting in improved quality of life, morbidity and even mortality in selected subgroups. However, precise criteria for selection of patients with respiratory muscle weakness who would benefit from treatment and the optimal methods for employing noninvasive positive pressure ventilation have yet to be clearly defined.

REFERENCES

1. Bourke SC, Gibson GJ. Sleep and breathing in neuromuscular disease. Eur Respir J 2002;19: 1194–201.

2. Guilleminault C, Shergill RP. Sleep-disordered breathing in neuromuscular disease. Curr Treat Options Neurol 2002;4:107–12.

3. Krachman SL, Criner GJ. Sleep and long-term ventilation. Respir Care Clin N Am 2002;8:611–29.

4. Shneerson JM. Respiration during sleep in neuromuscular and thoracic cage disorders. Monaldi Arch Chest Dis 2004;61:44–8.

5. Cirignotta F, Mondini S, Zucconi M, et al. Sleep-related breathing impairment in myotonic dystrophy. J Neurol 1987;235:80–5.

6. Smith PE, Calverley PM, Edwards RH, et al. Practical problems in the respiratory care of patients with muscular dystrophy. N Engl J Med 1987;316:1197–205.

7. Smith PE, Edwards RH, Calverley PM. Ventilation and breathing pattern during sleep in Duchenne muscular dystrophy. Chest 1989;96:1346–51.

8. Chokroverty S. Sleep-disordered breathing in neuromuscular disorders: a condition in search of recognition. Muscle Nerve 2001;24:451–5.

9. Bye PT, Ellis ER, Issa FG, et al. Respiratory failure and sleep in neuromuscular disease. Thorax 1990;45:241–7.

10. Gay PC, Westbrook PR, Daube JR, et al. Effects of alterations in pulmonary function and sleep variables on survival in patients with amyotrophic lateral sclerosis. Mayo Clin Proc 1991;66:686–94.

11. Howard RS, Wiles CM, Spencer GT. The late sequelae of poliomyelitis. Q J Med 1988;66:219–32.

12. Steljes DG, Kryger MH, Kirk BW, et al. Sleep in postpolio syndrome. Chest 1990;98:133–40.

13. Culebras A. Sleep and neuromuscular disorders. Neurol Clin 1996;14:791–805.

14. Labanowski M, Schmidt-Nowara W, Guilleminault C. Sleep and neuromuscular disease: frequency of sleep-disordered breathing in a neuromuscular disease clinic population. Neurology 1996;47:1173–80.

15. Guilleminault C, Philip P, Robinson A. Sleep and neuromuscular disease: bilevel positive airway pressure by nasal mask as a treatment for sleep disordered breathing in patients with neuromuscular disease. J Neurol Neurosurg Psychiatry 1998;65:225–32.

16. Chokroverty S. Physiologic changes in sleep. In: Chokroverty S, editor. Sleep disorders medicine: basic science, technical considerations and clinical aspects. 2nd edition. Boston: Butterworth-Heinemann; 1999. p. 95–126.

17. Worsnop C, Kay A, Pierce R, et al. Activity of respiratory pump and upper airway muscles during sleep onset. J Appl Physiol 1998;85:908–20.

18. Douglas NJ, White DP, Pickett CK, et al. Respiration during sleep in normal man. Thorax 1982;37:840–4.

19. Simon PM, Dempsey JA, Landry DM, et al. Effect of sleep on respiratory muscle activity during mechanical ventilation. Am Rev Respir Dis 1993;147:32–7.

20. Kay A, Trinder J, Kim Y. Progressive changes in airway resistance during sleep. J Appl Physiol 1996;81:282–92.

21. Berthon-Jones M, Sullivan CE. Ventilatory and arousal responses to hypoxia in sleeping humans. Am Rev Respir Dis 1982;125:632–9.

22. Douglas NJ, White DP, Weil JV, et al. Hypoxic ventilatory response decreases during sleep in normal men. Am Rev Respir Dis 1982;125:286–9.

23. Douglas NJ, White DP, Weil JV, et al. Hypercapnic ventilatory response in sleeping adults. Am Rev Respir Dis 1982;126:758–62.

24. Berthon-Jones M, Sullivan CE. Ventilation and arousal responses to hypercapnia in normal sleeping humans. J Appl Physiol 1984;57:59–67.

25. Tabachnik E, Muller NL, Bryan AC, et al. Changes in ventilation and chest wall mechanics during sleep in normal adolescents. J Appl Physiol 1981;51:557–64.

26. Gould GA, Gugger M, Molloy J, et al. Breathing pattern and eye movement density during REM sleep in humans. Am Rev Respir Dis 1988;138:874–7.

27. Millman RP, Knight H, Kline LR, et al. Changes in compartmental ventilation in association with eye movements during REM sleep. J Appl Physiol 1988;65:1196–202.

28. Schafer T, Schlafke ME. Respiratory changes associated with rapid eye movements in normo- and hypercapnia during sleep. J Appl Physiol 1998;85:2213–9.

29. Mier A. Respiratory muscle weakness. Respir Med 1990;84:351–9.

30. De Troyer A, Zegers De Beyl D, Thirion M. Function of the respiratory muscles in acute hemiplegia. Am Rev Respir Dis 1981;123:631–2.

31. Mier-Jedrzejowicz A, Green M. Respiratory muscle weakness associated with cerebellar atrophy. Am Rev Respir Dis 1988;137:673–7.

32. David WS, Bundlie SR, Mahdavi Z. Polysomnographic studies in amyotrophic lateral sclerosis. J Neurol Sci 1997;152(Suppl 1):S29–35.

33. Ferguson KA, Strong MJ, Ahmad D, et al. Sleep-disordered breathing in amyotrophic lateral sclerosis. Chest 1996;110:664–9.

34. Hukins CA, Hillman DR. Daytime predictors of sleep hypoventilation in Duchenne muscular dystrophy. Am J Respir Crit Care Med 2000;161:166–70.

35. Arnulf I, Similowski T, Salachas F, et al. Sleep disorders and diaphragmatic function in patients with amyotrophic lateral sclerosis. Am J Respir Crit Care Med 2000;161:849–56.

36. White JE, Drinnan MJ, Smithson AJ, et al. Respiratory muscle activity and oxygenation during sleep in patients with muscle weakness. Eur Respir J 1995;8:807–14.

37. De Troyer A, Heilporn A. Respiratory mechanics in quadriplegia. The respiratory function of the

intercostal muscles. Am Rev Respir Dis 1980;122: 591–600.

38. Estenne M, Heilporn A, Delhez L, et al. Chest wall stiffness in patients with chronic respiratory muscle weakness. Am Rev Respir Dis 1983;128:1002–7.

39. Gibson GJ, Pride NB, Davis JN, et al. Pulmonary mechanics in patients with respiratory muscle weakness. Am Rev Respir Dis 1977;115:389–95.

40. Khan Y, Heckmatt JZ. Obstructive apnoeas in Duchenne muscular dystrophy. Thorax 1994;49:157–61.

41. Smith PE, Calverley PM, Edwards RH. Hypoxemia during sleep in Duchenne muscular dystrophy. Am Rev Respir Dis 1988;137:884–8.

42. Chokroverty S. Sleep, breathing and neurologic disorders. In: Chokroverty S, editor. Sleep disorders medicine: basic science, technical considerations and clinical aspects. 2nd edition. Boston: Butterworth-Heinemann; 1999. p. 509–71.

43. Barbe F, Quera-Salva MA, McCann C, et al. Sleep-related respiratory disturbances in patients with Duchenne muscular dystrophy. Eur Respir J 1994; 7:1403–8.

44. Quera-Salva MA, Guilleminault C, Chevret S, et al. Breathing disorders during sleep in myasthenia gravis. Ann Neurol 1992;31:86–92.

45. Jubelt B, Agre JC. Characteristics and management of postpolio syndrome. JAMA 2000;284:412–4.

46. Laghi F, Tobin MJ. Disorders of the respiratory muscles. Am J Respir Crit Care Med 2003;168:10–48.

47. Cosgrove JL, Alexander MA, Kitts EL, et al. Late effects of poliomyelitis. Arch Phys Med Rehabil 1987; 68:4–7.

48. Attarian H. Sleep and neuromuscular disorders. Sleep Med 2000;1:3–9.

49. Guilleminault C, Motta J. Sleep apnea syndrome as as long term sequela of poliomyelitis. In: Guilleminault C, Dement WC, editors. Sleep apnea syndromes. New York: Alan R. Liss; 1978. p. 309–15.

50. Brown R. Amyotrophic lateral sclerosis. In: Gilman S, editor. Neurobase. 2nd edition. San Diego (CA): Arbor; 1999. p. 3–31.

51. Kimura K, Tachibana N, Kimura J, et al. Sleep-disordered breathing at an early stage of amyotrophic lateral sclerosis. J Neurol Sci 1999;164:37–43.

52. Minz M, Autret A, Laffont F, et al. A study on sleep in amyotrophic lateral sclerosis. Biomedicine 1979;30: 40–6.

53. Papazian O. Rapid eye movement sleep alterations in myasthenia gravis. Neurology 1976;26:311–6.

54. Amino A, Shiozawa Z, Nagasaka T, et al. Sleep apnoea in well-controlled myasthenia gravis and the effect of thymectomy. J Neurol 1998;245:77–80.

55. Patakas D, Tsara V, Zoglopitis F, et al. Nocturnal hypoxia in unilateral diaphragmatic paralysis. Respiration 1991;58:95–9.

56. Camfferman F, Bogaard JM, van der Meche FG, et al. Idiopathic bilateral diaphragmatic paralysis. Eur J Respir Dis 1985;67:65–71.

57. Mulvey DA, Aquilina RJ, Elliott MW, et al. Diaphragmatic dysfunction in neuralgic amyotrophy: an electrophysiologic evaluation of 16 patients presenting with dyspnea. Am Rev Respir Dis 1993; 147:66–71.

58. Skatrud J, Iber C, McHugh W, et al. Determinants of hypoventilation during wakefulness and sleep in diaphragmatic paralysis. Am Rev Respir Dis 1980; 121:587–93.

59. Finnimore AJ, Jackson RV, Morton A, et al. Sleep hypoxia in myotonic dystrophy and its correlation with awake respiratory function. Thorax 1994;49: 66–70.

60. Gilmartin JJ, Cooper BG, Griffiths CJ, et al. Breathing during sleep in patients with myotonic dystrophy and non-myotonic respiratory muscle weakness. Q J Med 1991;78:21–31.

61. Guilleminault C, Cummiskey J, Motta J, et al. Respiratory and hemodynamic study during wakefulness and sleep in myotonic dystrophy. Sleep 1978;1:19–31.

62. Ono S, Takahashi K, Jinnai K, et al. Loss of catecholaminergic neurons in the medullary reticular formation in myotonic dystrophy. Neurology 1998; 51:1121–4.

63. Veale D, Cooper BG, Gilmartin JJ, et al. Breathing pattern awake and asleep in patients with myotonic dystrophy. Eur Respir J 1995;8:815–8.

64. Ververs CC, Van der Meche FG, Verbraak AF, et al. Breathing pattern awake and asleep in myotonic dystrophy. Respiration 1996;63:1–7.

65. van Hilten JJ, Kerkhof GA, van Dijk JG, et al. Disruption of sleep-wake rhythmicity and daytime sleepiness in myotonic dystrophy. J Neurol Sci 1993;114:68–75.

66. van der Meche FG, Boogaard JM, van den Berg B. Treatment of hypersomnolence in myotonic dystrophy with a CNS stimulant. Muscle Nerve 1986;9: 341–4.

67. Phillips MF, Smith PE, Carroll N, et al. Nocturnal oxygenation and prognosis in Duchenne muscular dystrophy. Am J Respir Crit Care Med 1999;160: 198–202.

68. Segall D. Noninvasive nasal mask-assisted ventilation in respiratory failure of Duchenne muscular dystrophy. Chest 1988;93:1298–300.

69. Redding GJ, Okamoto GA, Guthrie RD, et al. Sleep patterns in nonambulatory boys with Duchenne muscular dystrophy. Arch Phys Med Rehabil 1985; 66:818–21.

70. Langevin B, Petitjean T, Philit F, et al. Nocturnal hypoventilation in chronic respiratory failure (CRF) due to neuromuscular disease. Sleep 2000; 23(Suppl 4):S204–8.

71. Braun NM, Arora NS, Rochester DF. Respiratory muscle and pulmonary function in polymyositis and other proximal myopathies. Thorax 1983;38:616–23.

72. Ragette R, Mellies U, Schwake C, et al. Patterns and predictors of sleep disordered breathing in primary myopathies. Thorax 2002;57:724–8.

73. Unterborn JN, Hill NS. Options for mechanical ventilation in neuromuscular diseases. Clin Chest Med 1994;15:765–81.

74. Bonsignore G, Marrone O, Macaluso C, et al. Validation of oximetry as a screening test for obstructive sleep apnoea syndrome. Eur Respir J Suppl 1990; 11:542s–4s.

75. Douglas NJ, Thomas S, Jan MA. Clinical value of polysomnography. Lancet 1992;339:347–50.

76. Meyer TJ, Eveloff SE, Kline LR, et al. One negative polysomnogram does not exclude obstructive sleep apnea. Chest 1993;103:756–60.

77. Williams AJ, Yu G, Santiago S, et al. Screening for sleep apnea using pulse oximetry and a clinical score. Chest 1991;100:631–5.

78. Barthlen GM. Nocturnal respiratory failure as an indication of noninvasive ventilation in the patient with neuromuscular disease. Respiration 1997; 64(Suppl 1):35–8.

79. Cerveri I, Fanfulla F, Zoia MC, et al. Sleep disorders in neuromuscular diseases. Monaldi Arch Chest Dis 1993;48:318–21.

80. Guilleminault C, Stoohs R, Clerk A, et al. A cause of excessive daytime sleepiness. The upper airway resistance syndrome. Chest 1993;104:781–7.

81. Bach JR, Penek J. Obstructive sleep apnea complicating negative-pressure ventilatory support in patients with chronic paralytic/restrictive ventilatory dysfunction. Chest 1991;99:1386–93.

82. Ellis ER, Bye PT, Bruderer JW, et al. Treatment of respiratory failure during sleep in patients with neuromuscular disease. Positive-pressure ventilation through a nose mask. Am Rev Respir Dis 1987;135:148–52.

83. Hill NS, Redline S, Carskadon MA, et al. Sleep-disordered breathing in patients with Duchenne muscular dystrophy using negative pressure ventilators. Chest 1992;102:1656–62.

84. Levy RD, Bradley TD, Newman SL, et al. Negative pressure ventilation. Effects on ventilation during sleep in normal subjects. Chest 1989;95:95–9.

85. Annane D, Quera-Salva MA, Lofaso F, et al. Mechanisms underlying effects of nocturnal ventilation on daytime blood gases in neuromuscular diseases. Eur Respir J 1999;13:157–62.

86. Barbe F, Quera-Salva MA, de Lattre J, et al. Long-term effects of nasal intermittent positive-pressure ventilation on pulmonary function and sleep architecture in patients with neuromuscular diseases. Chest 1996;110:1179–83.

87. Annane D, Orlikowski D, Chevret S, et al. Nocturnal mechanical ventilation for chronic hypoventilation in patients with neuromuscular and chest wall disorders. Cochrane Database Syst Rev 2007;4: CD001941.

88. Bach JR, Alba AS. Management of chronic alveolar hypoventilation by nasal ventilation. Chest 1990;97: 52–7.

89. Piper AJ, Sullivan CE. Effects of long-term nocturnal nasal ventilation on spontaneous breathing during sleep in neuromuscular and chest wall disorders. Eur Respir J 1996;9:1515–22.

90. Simonds AK, Elliott MW. Outcome of domiciliary nasal intermittent positive pressure ventilation in restrictive and obstructive disorders. Thorax 1995;50: 604–9.

91. Kleopa KA, Sherman M, Neal B, et al. Bipap improves survival and rate of pulmonary function decline in patients with ALS. J Neurol Sci 1999;164: 82–8.

92. Pinto AC, Evangelista T, Carvalho M, et al. Respiratory assistance with a non-invasive ventilator (Bipap) in MND/ALS patients: survival rates in a controlled trial. J Neurol Sci 1995;129(Suppl):19–26.

93. Lyall RA, Donaldson N, Fleming T, et al. A prospective study of quality of life in ALS patients treated with noninvasive ventilation. Neurology 2001;57: 153–6.

94. Clinical indications for noninvasive positive pressure ventilation in chronic respiratory failure due to restrictive lung disease, COPD, and nocturnal hypoventilation–a consensus conference report. Chest 1999;116:521–34.

95. Masa JF, Celli BR, Riesco JA, et al. Noninvasive positive pressure ventilation and not oxygen may prevent overt ventilatory failure in patients with chest wall diseases. Chest 1997;112:207–13.

96. MacDonald JR, Hill JD, Tarnopolsky MA. Modafinil reduces excessive somnolence and enhances mood in patients with myotonic dystrophy. Neurology 2002;59:1876–80.

97. Winkler G, Zifko U, Nader A, et al. Dose-dependent effects of inspiratory muscle training in neuromuscular disorders. Muscle Nerve 2000;23: 1257–60.

98. Mellies U, Ragette R, Schwake C, et al. Daytime predictors of sleep disordered breathing in children and adolescents with neuromuscular disorders. Neuromuscul Disord 2003;13:123–8.

Pulmonary Arterial Hypertension and Sleep

Namita Sood, MD

KEYWORDS

- Pulmonary hypertension • Sleep apnea
- Hypoxia-induced pulmonary hypertension

Pulmonary arterial hypertension (PAH) is defined as a mean pulmonary artery (PA) pressure greater than 25 mm Hg at rest or greater than 30 mm Hg with activity.[1] The common initial symptoms are dyspnea, fatigue, syncope, chest pain, or manifestations of right heart failure with lower extremity edema, ascites, and hepatomegaly.[2] PAH may be idiopathic (IPAH) or associated with connective tissue diseases, congenital heart disease, and exposure to exogenous factors including appetite suppressants or infectious agents such as HIV, and liver cirrhosis. Other secondary causes of PAH include disorders of the left ventricle (LV), chronic thromboembolic disease, and primary lung disease.[3] The evaluation of a patient with PAH entails a detailed work to define the etiology of the disease specifically ruling out LV systolic or diastolic dysfunction, or valvular disease by echocardiography, and hemodynamic measurement.[2]

HYPOXIA AND PULMONARY CIRCULATION

In chronic respiratory disease, hypoxia frequently occurs during the day and night. Hypoxia is known to cause an increase in pulmonary arterial pressure (PAP). This hypoxic vasoconstriction (HPV) is an important autoregulatory mechanism that diverts blood away from the underventilated alveoli and preserves the ventilation perfusion relationship. To survive oxygen deficiency, the cells activate a variety of adaptive mechanisms including inhibition of mRNA translation, which is a critical component of cell growth. These effects are mediated by hypoxia-inducible factors (HIF)-1α and HIF-2α that regulate most hypoxia-dependent genes and enable cells to adapt to hypoxia.

Hypoxia also triggers several other mechanisms that interface with HIF signaling. Recently it has been shown that hypoxia induces the synthesis of mRNA some of which protect against apoptosis. A set of mRNA modulate expression of vascular endothelial growth factor, a principal growth factor for endothelial cells, and other angiogenic factors.[4–6]

An acute decrease in oxygen concentration induces a reversible constriction of vascular smooth muscle of the preacinar smooth muscles. This leads to an increase of approximately 4–8 mm Hg in the PA pressure and an increase in pulmonary vascular resistance (PVR). Upon restoration of normoxia, the PVR returns to normal.[7,8] Chronic hypoxia may lead to PAH. Hypoxia-induced PAH is usually mild and theoretically should be reversible upon correction of hypoxia. Rodents exposed to chronic hypoxia develop proliferation of cells of all three layers of the pulmonary vessel: the endothelium, pulmonary artery smooth muscle cell (PASMC), and the adventitial fibroblasts.[6] This vascular remodeling noted with chronic hypoxia is not completely understood; several mechanisms have been implicated. Endothelial dysfunction is noted; there is an imbalance in vasodilators and vasoconstrictors produced by the endothelium. Increased levels of endothelin-1, a potent vasoconstrictor, cell mitogen, and a proinflammatory peptide are found in hypoxic animals.[9] Prostacyclins, potent vasodilators, play a role in the development of hypoxia-induced PAH. Overexpression of the prostacyclin synthase, an enzyme responsible for prostacyclin production in mice exposed to hypoxia, protected them from development of pulmonary hypertension.[10,11]

Serotonin (5-HT) has been implicated in hypoxia-related PAH. 5-HT promotes vasoconstriction and

The Ohio State University Medical Center, University Hospital, James Cancer Hospital, 201 Davis Heart and Lung Research Institute, 473 West 12th Avenue, Columbus, OH 43210, USA
E-mail address: namita.sood@osumc.edu

Sleep Med Clin 3 (2008) 551–556
doi:10.1016/j.jsmc.2008.08.004
1556-407X/08/$ – see front matter

vascular smooth muscle growth. 5-HT exerts its vasoactive properties via transporter 5-HTT and receptors 5-HTA1, 5-HTA2, 5-HTB1, and 5-HTB2. Animals lacking the 5-HT transporter gene are protected against hypoxic PAH.[12] Patients with chronic obstructive pulmonary disease (COPD) who had the LL genotype (which is associated with higher levels of 5-HTT expression in PASMC) had more severe PAH than the SS genotype or heterozygotes.[13]

The mitochondria of the PASMC appear to play a key role in HPV. Upon exposure to hypoxia, the mitochondrial reactive oxygen species (ROS) production decreases. This inhibits the oxygen-sensitive ATP-dependent voltage–gated K+ (Kv) channel and causes membrane depolarization and activation of voltage-gated L-type calcium channels. This is followed by calcium influx that triggers calmodulin-mediated activation of myosin light kinase, actin–myosin interaction, contraction, and initiates HPV. HIF-1α activation downregulates oxygen-sensitive Kv channels and initiates a cascade that leads to enhanced vasoconstriction.[14,15]

Rho kinase is a small GTPase which has been implicated in the formation of stress fibers and focal adhesions, cell morphology, and smooth muscle contraction. It regulates the phosphorylation of myosin light chain smooth muscle contraction and stress fiber formation in nonmuscle cells. Rho kinase inhibitor prevented development of PAH in hypoxic mice.[16,17] In addition, platelet-derived growth factor (PDGF) which is a potent mitogen of pulmonary smooth muscles may play a role. It has been shown that blocking the PDGF receptor reversed hypoxia-induced PAH in mice.[18] Endothelin-1 may also contribute to the inhibition of Kv channel expression.[19]

Hypoxia also leads to an influx of neutrophils and macrophages in the perivascular spaces. There is induction of the proinflammatory cytokines and chemokines such as monocyte chemoattractant protein MCP-1, macrophage inflammatory protein MIP-2 interleukin (IL)-1β, and IL-6.[20]

Pulmonary Arterial Hypertension in Obstructive Sleep Apne

In obstructive sleep apnea (OSA), hypoxia may be limited to the sleep period. This raises the question whether nocturnal hypoxia is enough to cause PAH. Rats treated with alternating periods of normoxia and hypercapnic hypoxia every 30 seconds for eight hours a day, five days per week, for five weeks developed significant increases in PA pressures and increased right ventricular (RV) weight and hematocrit.[21]

Patients with OSA have been found to have increased sympathetic activity.[22] They generate significant negative intrathoracic pressure by repetitive diaphragmatic effort against an occluded upper airway. This negative pressure has a direct effect on the heart. It leads to an increased transmyocardial pressure gradient which increases cardiac afterload, venous return, and a leftward shift of the intracardiac septum.[23] There is evidence of endothelial dysfunction; endothelin-1 has been shown to be increased. There is decreased nitric oxide bioavailability measured by nitrite–nitrate concentrations which improves with treatment of OSA.[24,25] Increased levels of markers of inflammation such as C-reactive protein and IL-6 are noted. There is increased expression of adhesion molecules in monocytes. Total serum fibrinogen and whole blood viscosity levels are elevated in OSA. There is increased platelet activation and aggregation, and reduced fibrinolytic activity; plasminogen activator inhibitor is elevated.[26–29]

However, not all patients with OSA develop PAH. The prevalence of pulmonary hypertension in patients with sleep apnea has been reported to vary from 9% to 48%. The true prevalence is unclear simply because different methods have been used to define PAH. Many of these studies are retrospective or small prospective cohort studies. Some have included patients with obesity hypoventilation; and patients with cardiac and lung disease were not always excluded. Apprill and colleagues[30] studied 46 patients with OSA and found nine (20 %) to have PAH. Patients with PAH tended to have lower Pao_2, higher $Paco_2$, lower forced vital capacity (FVC), and lower forced expired volume in one second (FEV_1). The presence of PAH did not correlate with the apnea-hypopnea index (AHI). PAH was associated with the presence of COPD and severe obesity. The investigators did not mention the pulmonary capillary wedge pressure or LV end-diastolic pressure. Laks and colleagues[31] studied 100 patients with AHI greater than 20 per hour; patients with other medical diseases were excluded. When awake, 42% of them had a mean PAP (mPAP) greater than 20 mm Hg and 6% had a MPAP greater than 80 mm Hg. The patients with PAH tended to have lower Pao_2 and FEV_1, and higher $Paco_2$. Another prospective study[32] of 114 consecutive patients found that 19% of sleep apnea patients had PAP greater than or equal to 20mm Hg; patients with COPD were not excluded. Podzuz and colleagues[33] measured PA pressures in 65 patients with OSA at rest and during exercise. Thirteen had PAH at rest and another 31 were noted to have increased PA pressures with exercise. Eight of these patients had other underlying cardio-pulmonary disease. Eleven of the 65 had severe sleep apnea. Six of these 11 patients had a moderate increase in PA pressures during sleep. Five had a severe increase in PA pressures with accompanied increase in the cardiac output and pulmonary capillary wedge pressure suggesting an element of LV dysfunction. Bady and colleagues[34] performed right heart catheterization in 44 patients with OSA. Twelve out of 44 (27%) had MPAP greater than 20 mm Hg with normal wedge pressures. The patients with increased PA pressures tended to have lower daytime Pao_2, higher $Paco_2$, more severe nocturnal hypoxia, and higher body mass index (BMI). Another study undertaken by Chaoaut and Wietzenblum[35] included 222 patients with AHI greater than 20, and 37 (17%) of the patients had MPAP greater than 20 mm Hg. The patients with PAH tended to have lower Pao_2, lower FVC, and higher BMI. Kesseler and Chaouat[36] found that among 181 patients with pure sleep apnea, only 9% had mild PAH with MPAP greater than 20 mm Hg; whereas 59% of the 27 patients with obesity hypoventilation had MPAP greater than 20 mm Hg. Sajkov and colleagues[37,38] studied 27 patients without underlying lung and cardiac disease and found 11 to have MPAP of 26mm Hg. There was no difference in the AHI, BMI, or lung function. However, the patients with PAH were more hypoxic during the day which could be the cause or the result of PAH.

Taken together, these data suggest that the frequency of PAH in patients with simple OSA is low and the PAH is often mild. OSA patients who develop PAH tend to be older, heavier, more hypoxic, and have worse lung function. There are clearly patients who have OSA and severe elevation of PAP with their pulmonary hemodynamics mimicking those seen in patients with IPAH. What role the hypoxia associated with OSA plays in the development of severe PAH is not known. Genetic susceptibility factors that may predispose certain patients to develop significant PAH need to be studied. Patients with OSA frequently suffer from hypertension and the LV dysfunction has not always been properly evaluated in these studies. The presence of other pulmonary disease in conjunction with OSA seems to be a mediating factor in the development of PAH.

There are reports of improvement of PAP following treatment of sleep apnea following tracheostomy. Alchanatis studied 29 patients with OSA using Doppler echocardiography before and after treatment with continuous positive airway pressure (CPAP).[39,40] Twenty percent of patients with OSA had mild PAH. Six months of treatment with CPAP resulted in modest reductions in the PAP

(25.6 $\pm$ 4 to 19.5 mm Hg). Sajkov and colleagues treated 20 patients with OSA for four months using CPAP. CPAP therapy reduced the PAP and improved hypoxic pulmonary vascular reactivity. A more recent placebo controlled trial included 23 OSA patients. PAH was defined as PAP greater than 30 mm Hg by echocardiogram and 10 OSA patients met the definition of PAH at baseline. All patients were treated with CPAP or sham CPAP in a randomized crossover design. CPAP therapy reduced PA systolic pressure significantly after 4 months; more so in those with PAH and evidence of LV diastolic dysfunction at baseline.[41]

It needs to be noted that all these studies use echocardiogram as a tool to assess PAH and cannot totally exclude left ventricular dysfunction, which may contribute to PH. The PH in patients with sleep apnea is typically mild and may be more responsive to correction of hypoxia. Prolonged hypoxia may lead to remodeling of the pulmonary vessels by the mechanisms described above and result in significant increases in PAP and RV failure. If this occurs, the process may not be completely reversible by correction of nocturnal hypoxia.

PULMONARY HYPERTENSION AND OVERLAP SYNDROME

Sleep apnea and COPD are both common conditions and they may coexist (overlap syndrome). Patients with overlap syndrome tend to have greater oxygen desaturations with sleep than patients with COPD alone with the same degree of airway obstruction. The prevalence of PAH is higher in this subgroup and they are at a higher risk for developing hypercapnic respiratory failure. Chaouat and Wietzenblum[42] noted that in 26 patients with sleep apnea who had a MPAP greater than 20 mm Hg, the prevalence of PAH was 36% in patients with the overlap syndrome and 9% for those with obesity hyperventilation alone. Patients with the overlap syndrome may develop PAH even in the absence of significant airway obstruction. Bradley and colleagues[43,44] noted that patients with OSA who had evidence of bronchial obstruction tended to have greater degree of hypoxemia-hypercapnia and evidence of right heart failure even though the degree of obstruction was mild. The COPD likely plays a role in the development of PAH but it is important to emphasize that the degree of obstruction is frequently mild.

SLEEP DISORDERS IN PATIENTS WITH PULMONARY ARTERIAL HYPERTENSION

It is common for patients with chronic lung disease to have sleep-disordered breathing. Patients with

IPAH frequently have increased Alveolar-arterial (A-a) gradient and have oxygen desaturation with activity such as a six-minute walk. The majority of these patients will have nocturnal desaturations. In a small study of 13 patients with IPAH who underwent a standard polysomnogram, all patients had normal apnea indexes and two had mild hypopneas. The authors defined significant desaturations as greater than10% of total sleep time with an oxygen saturation less than 90%. Ten (77%) had nocturnal desaturations and these were associated with lower FEV_1 values, lower oxygenation status, and higher A-a gradient. There was no difference in the BMI, six-minute walk distance, or PA pressure between those with or without nocturnal destaurations.[45] Minai and colleagues[46] studied 43 patients with IPAH of whom 30 patients (69%) had nocturnal desaturations. In this study, the patients who desaturated tended to have worse disease and RV function. The patients who desaturated were also older. More than half of the patients who had nocturnal desaturations during sleep did not have desaturations with activity. Based on these data, nocturnal desaturations tend to be quite frequent in patients with IPAH and may be unrecognized. Routine overnight pulse oximetry is recommended in patients evaluated for PAH.

Patients with IPAH have significant limitations in their activity and may suffer from anxiety and depression from chronic illness. They frequently exhibit poor sleep hygiene and poor sleep due to anxiety. Restless leg syndrome may occur in these patients. A detailed history for sleep related disorders should be obtained from patients with PAH. Patients who have significant oxygen desaturations at night or have physical examination findings that raise the possibility OSA should undergo a full sleep study.

SUMMARY

Despite the evidence that hypoxia in animals leads to irreversible changes in the pulmonary vasculature, the incidence of severe PAH in patients with isolated OSA is not that frequent. However, patients with concomitant airway obstruction and obesity hypoventilation are at high risk for developing significant PAH. Patients who have persistent hypoxia or symptoms after optimal therapy for OSA has been instituted should be evaluated for PAH. The role of selective vasodilator therapies currently approved for PAH in this setting is not known. It is likely that the mild PAH noted in these patients will improve with optimal treatment of OSA. Use of selective vasodilators in patients with underlying lung disease may cause worsening ventilation-perfusion matching and lead to worsening hypoxia. More important, LV systolic and diastolic dysfunctions are quite frequent in patients with OSA. These treatments have not shown to be of benefit in patients with LV dysfunction and associated PAH. There are no long-term studies to define the natural progression of PAH in these patients and its impact on quality of life. There may be benefit from current therapies in patients who have severe elevation of their PAP despite adequate treatment of OSA but this has not been studied.

Future studies need to systematically evaluate these patients using standard criteria to define OSA and PAH. The impact of coexistent disease and genetic susceptibility on development of PAH and its natural course needs to be defined.

REFERENCES

1. Gaine SP, Rubin LJ. Primary pulmonary hypertension. Lancet 1998;352:719–29.
2. McGoon M, Gutterman D, et al. Screening, early detection and diagnosis of pulmonary arterial hypertension. Chest 2004;126:14S–34S.
3. Simmonneau G, Galie N, et al. Clinical classification of pulmonary hypertension. J Am Coll Cardiol 2004; 43:5S–12S.
4. Liu L, Cash TP, Jones RG, et al. Hypoxia-induced energy stress regulates mRNA translation and cell growth. Mol Cell 2006;21:521–31.
5. Kulshreshtha R, Ferracin M, Negrini M, et al. Regulation of microRNA expression: the hypoxic component. Cell Cycle 2007;12:1426–31.
6. Voelkel NF, Tuder RM. Hypoxia-induced pulmonary vascular remodeling—a model for what human disease? J Clin Invest 2000;106:733–8.
7. Archer SL, McMurtry IF, Weir EK. Mechanisms of acute hypoxic and hyperoxic changes in pulmonary vascular reactivity. In: Weir EK, Reeves JT, editors. Pulmonary vascular physiology and pathophysiology. New York: Marcel Dekker Inc.; 1989. p. 241–90.
8. Peng W, Hoidal JR. Role of novel KCa opener in regulating K+ channels of hypoxic human pulmonary vascular cells. Am J Respir Cell Mol Biol 1999;20: 737–45.
9. Elton TS, Oparil S, et al. Normobaric hypoxia stimulates endothelin-1 gene expression in the rat. Am J Physiol Regul Integr Comp Physiol 1992;263:R1260–4.
10. Voelkel NF, Margonroth M. Potential role of arachidonic acid metabolites in hypoxic pulmonary vasoconstriction. Chest 1997;111:1622–30.
11. Geraci MW, Gao B. Pulmonary prostacyclin synthase overexpression in transgenic mice protects against development of hypoxic pulmonary hypertension. J Clin Invest 1999;103:1509–15.

12. Eddahibi S, Hanoun N, et al. Attenuated hypoxic pulmonary hypertension in mice lacking the 5-hyoxytryptamine transporter gene. J Clin Invest 2000;11:1555–62.

13. Eddahibi S, Raffesentin B, et al. Polyorphism of serotonin transporter gene and pulmonary hypertension in chronic obstructive lung disease. Circulation 2003;108:1839–44.

14. Reeve HL, Archer SL, et al. Ion channels in pulmonary vasculature. Pulm Pharmacol Ther 1997;10:243–52.

15. McMurtry MS, Archer SL, et al. Gene therapy targeting survivin selectively induces pulmonary vascular apoptosis and reverse pulmonary arterial hypertension. J Clin Invest 2005;6:1479–91.

16. Broughton BS, Walker BR, et al. Chronic hypoxia induces Rho kinase-dependent myogenic tone in small vessels. Am J Physiol Lung Cell Mol Physiol 2008;294:L797–806.

17. Fagan KA, Oka M, et al. Attenuation of acute hypoxic pulmonary vasoconstriction and hypoxic pulmonary hypertension by inhibition of Rho kinase. Am J Physiol Lung Cell Mol Physiol 2004;287:L656–64.

18. Schemuly T, Dony E, et al. Reversal of experimental pulmonary hypertension by PDGF inhibition. J Clin Invest 2005;115:2811–21.

19. Whitman EM, Pisarcik S, et al. Endothelin-1 mediates hypoxia-induced inhibition of voltage gated K+ channel expression in pulmonary arterial myocytes. Am J Physiol Lung Cell Mol Physiol 2007;294:L309–18.

20. Wood JG, Johnson JS, et al. Systemic hypoxia increases leukocyte emigration and vascular permeability in conscious rats. J Appl Physiol 2000;89:1561–9.

21. McGuire M, Bradford A. Chronic intermittent hypercapnic hypoxia increases pulmonary arterial pressure and hematocrit in rats. Eur Respir J 2001;18:279–85.

22. Somers VK, Dyken ME, et al. Sympathetic neural mechanisms in obstructive sleep apnea. J Clin Invest 1995;96:1897–904.

23. Shiomi T, Guilleminault AS, et al. Leftward shift of the intraventricular septum and pulsus paradoxus in obstructive sleep apnea. Chest 1991;100:894–902.

24. Philips BG, Narkrawicz K, et al. Effects of obstructive sleep apnea on endothelin-1 and blood pressure. J Hypertens 1999;17:61–6.

25. Lavie L, Hefetz F, et al. Plasma levels of nitric oxide and L-arginine in sleep apnea patients: effects of sleep apnea treatment. J Mol Neurosci 2003;21:57–64.

26. Shamsuzzaman AS, Winnicki M, et al. C-reactive protein in patients with obstructive sleep apnea. Circulation 2002;105:2462–4.

27. Yokoe T, Minoguchi K, et al. Elevated levels of C-reactive protein and interleukin-6 in patients with obstructive sleep apnea are reduced by nasal continues pressure. Circulation 2003;107:1129–34.

28. Bokinsky G, Miller M, et al. Spontaneous platelet activation and aggregation during obstructive sleep apnea and its response to therapy with nasal continuous positive airway pressure—a preliminary investigation. Chest 1995;108:625–30.

29. Chin K, Ohi M, et al. Effects of NCPAP therapy on fibrinogen levels in obstructive sleep apnea. Am J Respir Crit Care Med 1996;153:1972–6.

30. Apprill M, Weitzenblum E, et al. Frequency and mechanism of daytime pulmonary hypertension in patients with obstructive sleep apnea. Cor Vasa 1991;33:42–9.

31. Laks L, Lehrhaft B, et al. Pulmonary hypertension in obstructive sleep apnea. Eur Respir J 1999;8:537–41.

32. Krieger J, Sforza E, et al. Pulmonary hypertension, hypoxia, and hypercapnia in obstructive sleep apnea patients. Chest 1989;96:729–37.

33. Podzuz T, Bauer W, et al. Sleep apnea and pulmonary hypertension. Klin Wochenschr 1986;64:131–4.

34. Bady E, Achkar A, et al. Pulmonary arterial hypertension in patients with sleep apnea syndrome. Thorax 2000;55:934–9.

35. Chaouat A, Wietzenblum E. Pulmonary hemodynamics in obstructive sleep apnea syndrome: results in 220 consecutive patients. Chest 1996;109:380–6.

36. Kessler R, Chaouat A, et al. The obesity-hypoventilation syndrome revisited: a prospective study of 34 consecutive cases. Chest 2001;120:369–76.

37. Sajkov D, Wang T, et al. Pulmonary hemodynamics in patients with obstructive sleep apnea without lung disease. Am J Respir Crit Care Med 1999;159:1518–26.

38. Motta J, Guilleminault C, et al. Tracheostomy and hemodynamic changes in sleep-induced apnea. Ann Intern Med 1978;89:454–8.

39. Alchanatis M, Toukohoriti G, et al. Daytime pulmonary hypertension in patients with obstructive sleep apnea. Respiration 2001;68:566–72.

40. Sajkov D, Wang T, et al. Continuous positive airway pressure treatment improves pulmonary hemodynamics in patients with obstructive sleep apnea. Am J Respir Crit Care Med 2002;165:152–8.

41. Arias MA, Garcia-Rio F, et al. Pulmonary hypertension in obstructive sleep apnea: effects of continuous positive airway pressure: a randomized, controlled crossover study. Eur Heart J 2006;27:1106–13.

42. Chaouat A, Wietzenblum E. Association of chronic obstructive lung disease and sleep apnea syndrome. Am Rev Respir Dis 1995;151:82–6.

43. Bradley TD, Rutherford A, et al. Role of daytime hypoxemia in the pathogenesis of right heart failure in

obstructive sleep apnea syndrome. Am Rev Respir Dis 1985;131:835–9.

44. Bradley TD, Rutherford A, et al. Role of diffuse airway obstruction in the hypercapnia of obstructive apnea. Am Rev Respir Dis 1986;134:920–4.

45. Rafanan AL, Golish JA, et al. Nocturnal hypoxemia is common in primary pulmonary hypertension. Chest 2001;120:894–9.

46. Minai OA, Pandya CM, et al. Predictors of nocturnal oxygen desaturations in pulmonary arterial hypertension. Chest 2007;131:109–17.

Chronic Noninvasive Positive-Pressure Ventilation: Considerations During Sleep

Murtuza M. Ahmed, MD*, Richard J. Schwab, MD

KEYWORDS

- Noninvasive ventilation • Sleep • REM
- Obesity hypoventilation syndrome
- Chronic obstructive pulmonary disease
- Management • Treatment • Side effects • Review

Over the last 2 decades, noninvasive ventilation (NIV) has become a proven and accepted treatment for hypoxic and hypercapnic respiratory failure from a variety of underlying causes.[1,2] Respiratory failure, regardless of the cause, leads to diminished quality of life and decreased survival.[3–5] Application of NIV can improve numerous physiologic parameters and gas exchange abnormalities, as has been well documented in studies of both acute and chronic respiratory failure.[6–16] In most instances of chronic respiratory failure, NIV is applied at night during the sleeping hours, when the respiratory status of a patient is most vulnerable. However, there is relatively little data on how this intervention affects sleep itself. This review highlights the physiologic effects of NIV applied during the sleeping hours, examines its sleep-state effects in several important disease entities, and reviews patient selection criteria and methods of instituting NIV.

VENTILATION DURING SLEEP IN THE NORMAL HOST

The most challenging period of the circadian cycle with regards to ventilation is in sleep. During sleep, numerous physiologic changes take place in the normal host. These changes increase the work of breathing. In the individual with chronic respiratory illness, this challenge is magnified in proportion to the degree of disease severity. Body position, control of breathing, airway resistance, and activation of the respiratory pump muscles are all altered during sleep as compared with wakefulness.[17,18]

Sleep induces several significant changes in breathing in the normal subject. A sleeping individual experiences a 20% decline in tidal volumes.[19–23] While the respiratory rate during sleep increases slightly to make up for this loss, there is still a 10% to 15% decrease in minute ventilation.[19–23] As a result of these sleep-induced changes, Pa_{CO_2} rises 3 to 7 mm Hg, while the Pa_{O_2} may fall from 4 to 9 mm Hg; oxygen saturations may decline by 2%.[20,21] Central chemoreceptor response to the hypercapnia and hypoxia associated with these physiologic changes during sleep is also blunted, more so during rapid eye movement (REM) sleep.[24–26] The sleeping individual is not able to mount an adequate ventilatory response that would fully compensate for these physiologic perturbations. This is most evident during REM sleep, when the output from accessory respiratory muscles is essentially absent and only the diaphragm remains active in maintaining the work of breathing. Furthermore, respiratory drive is decreased during REM sleep, relative to non-REM and wake states.[18]

Center for Sleep and Respiratory Neurobiology, University of Pennsylvania School of Medicine, Translational Research Laboratories, Suite 2100, 125 S. 31st Street, Philadelphia, PA 19104, USA
* Corresponding author.
E-mail address: murtuza.ahmed@uphs.upenn.edu (M.M. Ahmed).

Sleep Med Clin 3 (2008) 557–568
doi:10.1016/j.jsmc.2008.08.002
1556-407X/08/$ – see front matter. Published by Elsevier Inc.

During sleep, upper airway muscle tone changes, resulting in increased upper airway resistance.[27,28] This has been shown to occur at the level of the geniohyoid muscle[29] and tensor palatini muscle.[28] Lower airway resistance appears to have a circadian cycle and tends to increase during the night hours. In healthy individuals, peak expiratory flow rates may diminish as much as 8% during sleep compared with daytime values.[30]

Cardiovascular changes are also prominent during sleep. Most notably, blood pressure decreases by 10% to 15% during non-REM sleep. Cardiac output, stroke volume, and heart rate also decrease.[31,32] Heart rate, cardiac output, and blood pressure during sleep differ from those during the wake state.[31,32]

VENTILATION DURING SLEEP IN THE COMPROMISED HOST

While these state-dependent physiologic changes may not pose a significant problem for normal individuals, those with respiratory compromise have a much more difficult time during the sleeping hours. As a result, in patients with borderline oxygenation, maintaining adequate oxyhemoglobin saturations becomes increasingly difficult while asleep. Moreover, these individuals may be operating at the edge of the steep shoulder on the oxyhemoglobin-dissociation curve while awake. In the sleep state, even a small decrement in Pa_{O_2} may therefore correspond to a very large decline in oxygen saturation. In patients with hyperinflation, altered length–tension relationships at the level of the diaphragm further impair pulmonary mechanics, thereby exacerbating the gas exchange abnormalities associated with sleep.[33]

Patients with compromised ventilatory pump function, most commonly from neuromuscular disease, may have impairments in their ability to increase their respiratory rate or have a more pronounced decline in the activity of accessory muscles while asleep, further compromising their ventilation.[34] Nocturnal respiratory impairment in these patients is largely a function of the location of disease. In individuals with accessory muscle or diaphragmatic weakness, hypoventilation is likely to occur.[34] In those with upper airway weakness, sleep-disordered breathing is common.[35–37] Altered chest wall mechanics found in thoracic cage abnormalities (such as kyphoscoliosis) lead to increased work of breathing and an increased tendency for respiratory muscle fatigue due to the mechanical disadvantage.[18,33,34] During sleep, patients with thoracic cage abnormalities may develop hypoventilation, as these patients are more dependent on input from accessory muscles.

The resulting decrease in functional residual capacity leads to ventilation/perfusion mismatch, causing hypoxia.[38]

Beyond these abnormalities in lung mechanics, sleep itself is often altered in individuals with respiratory dysfunction. Patients with chronic respiratory failure from obstructive or restrictive causes have reductions in total sleep time and sleep efficiency compared with healthy individuals.[39,40] Stages 3 and 4 sleep, along with REM sleep, appear to be preserved,[39,40] although one study noted that subjects with both hypoxia and ventilatory compromise had reductions in REM.[41] Stages 1 and 2 sleep also appear to be disturbed by respiratory dysfunction, although this has been less well studied.[17]

While NIV improves nocturnal Pa_{CO_2} and Pa_{O_2} while also reducing the work of breathing in compromised individuals, relatively little is known regarding its effects on sleep and sleep quality (see section on effect of NIV on sleep parameters below).

PHYSIOLOGIC CHANGES INDUCED BY NONINVASIVE VENTILATION

NIV has been shown to effectively treat chronic respiratory failure from a variety of conditions, including neuromuscular disorders, diaphragmatic dysfunction, chest wall deformities, and chronic lung disease processes (**Box 1**).[1,42,43]

Box 1
Sources of chronic respiratory failure treated by NIV

Alveolar hypoventilation syndromes

Neuromuscular disease

Amyotrophic lateral sclerosis

Duchenne muscular dystrophy

Postpolio syndrome

Multiple sclerosis

Myasthenia gravis

Guillain-Barré syndrome

High spinal cord injury

Bilateral diaphragm paralysis

Kyphoscoliosis and chest wall deformities

Restrictive lung disease

Cystic fibrosis

Obesity-hypoventilation syndrome (Pickwickian syndrome)

Central sleep apnea

Chronic obstructive pulmonary disease

With the extensive experience developed using negative-pressure NIV during the polio epidemics, investigators have shown that negative-pressure NIV improves gas exchange and decreases patient symptoms.[44–46] Moreover, these improvements were sustained over a period of many years of use, with excellent long-term survival in patients with respiratory failure from a variety of causes.[44–46] While negative-pressure ventilation was used successfully in the past, it has been largely supplanted by positive-pressure ventilation techniques. The major disadvantages of negative-pressure ventilation include the necessity to lie in the supine position, resulting in back and shoulder pain, and the potential hazard of precipitating upper airway collapse and obstructive apneas in some individuals, particularly during REM sleep.[47] Therefore, before instituting negative-pressure NIV therapy, patients should undergo polysomnography while using negative-pressure NIV to rule out sleep apnea. Initiation of negative-pressure NIV can be time consuming and the devices are not portable. As a result of these limitations, negative-pressure NIV has largely been supplanted by positive-pressure ventilation. This review therefore focuses on studies that have been conducted using noninvasive positive-pressure ventilation and uses the abbreviation NIV to refer to noninvasive positive-pressure ventilation, unless otherwise indicated.

The physiologic benefits of nocturnal NIV use in individuals with chronic respiratory failure appear to carry over into the following day. Windisch and colleagues[15] recently examined the daytime consequences of nocturnal NIV in a group of 12 subjects and controls with stable, chronic respiratory failure. As expected, those subjects on NIV had lower $Paco_2$ levels immediately following cessation of NIV. However, the investigators also found that the effects of NIV persisted into the daytime hours, lasting for at least 3 hours and as many as 15 hours during spontaneous breathing. A concomitant increase in tidal volume was also noted, while respiratory rates remained stable. These findings were not present in controls. Other investigators have demonstrated similar results. Using a series of consecutive patients with stable chronic respiratory failure, Schönhofer and colleagues[48] demonstrated that, in addition to decreasing daytime $Paco_2$ values, nocturnal NIV also improved tidal volume in patients. These beneficial physiologic findings were confirmed in a randomized crossover trial with chronic obstructive pulmonary disease (COPD) patients by Diaz and colleagues,[49] in which subjects were placed on either NIV or sham. Beyond these physiologic parameters, subjects on active nocturnal NIV also reported improvements in daytime alertness and decreases in sleepiness and respiratory symptom scores.

In summary, chronic nocturnal NIV has numerous benefits that have been demonstrated over the last 2 decades. These include improvements in gas exchange, correction of hypercapnia and hypoxia, subsequent gas exchange improvements that carry over into the daytime, reduction in sleep fragmentation and nocturnal awakenings, respiratory muscle rest, improvement in daytime symptoms of hypoxia and hypercapnia, and improvement in symptoms of congestive heart failure.[50]

EFFECTS OF NONINVASIVE VENTILATION ON SLEEP PARAMETERS

While the benefits of NIV vis-à-vis gas exchange and pulmonary function have been extensively investigated, the impact of NIV on sleep is less clear. Few studies have examined the effect of NIV on sleep quality and architecture. Nonetheless, the preponderance of data suggests that NIV improves sleep quality and duration in patients with chronic respiratory failure from a variety of causes.[17]

The effect of NIV in patients with cystic fibrosis has recently been the subject of a Cochrane review by Moran and colleagues.[51] These investigators included data from seven clinical trials[10,52–57] in their pooled analysis and examined the impact of NIV on such outcomes as nocturnal gas exchange and sleep parameters. They noted that NIV can be useful as an airway clearance tool and may also improve nocturnal gas exchange during sleep.[51] However, with regard to sleep quality and architecture, the investigators found little evidence of benefit in the trials they reviewed.[51] Specifically, Gozal did not find a difference in either total sleep time, REM sleep time, or sleep latency among the cystic fibrosis group treated with NIV versus those on either oxygen or room air.[10] Milross and colleagues[55] also did not find differences in any of these sleep variables. A more recent clinical trial by Young and coworkers[57] of nine adult cystic fibrosis patients also failed to demonstrate appreciable differences in sleep architecture or daytime sleepiness (as measured by the Epworth sleepiness score) with NIV. Nonetheless, they did find that subjects using NIV had improved exercise capacity and nocturnal gas exchange compared with baseline and those on oxygen.[57]

In other patient populations, sleep does appear to be improved with NIV. Teschler and colleagues[58] found that in their heterogeneous group of patients with chronic respiratory failure, sealing the mouth while using NIV resulted in improved REM and a trend toward increased delta sleep. Barbé's group studied 7 subjects with neuromuscular disease before and after initiation of NIV.[59] After 18 months of treatment, the subjects had improvements in sleep efficiency (59% versus 83%, $P < .05$) and the amount of delta sleep also doubled (8% versus 16%, $P < .05$).[59] Annane and colleagues[6] also found improvements after 1 year of NIV use in a group of 14 patients with restrictive thoracic disease in both sleep efficiency (74% at baseline versus 87% at 1 year, $P < .01$) and delta sleep (11% at baseline versus 20% at 1 year, $P < .05$). More convincingly, follow-up polysomnography at 3 years demonstrated that these improvements were maintained.

Other lines of evidence for improved sleep and quality of life with NIV come from studies of treatment withdrawal.[12,60,61] As expected, in these studies, withdrawal of NIV resulted in increased nocturnal P_{CO_2} and decreased nocturnal oxygen saturation. However, these patients also had decreased sleep efficiency, total sleep time, delta sleep, and REM sleep,[61] as well as more arousals.[12] They also reported worse sleep quality, daytime hypersomnolence, and morning headaches while off NIV.[60] Resumption of therapy reversed these changes.[12,61]

There are relatively few studies comparing NIV to tracheostomy. Bach and colleagues[62] described their experience with long-term NIV compared with patients who underwent tracheostomy. While NIV was generally thought of as more comfortable, those who underwent tracheostomy reported better sleep quality and a better sense of security. Other studies surveying subjects with either chronic NIV or tracheostomies have found that both groups had similar quality-of-life assessments,[63,64] although no objective sleep data were measured in these studies.

A recently published Cochrane review by Annane and others[65] reviewed clinical trials using NIV to treat respiratory failure in patients with neuromuscular disease and chest wall disorders. Unfortunately, of the large number of published studies, very few met their inclusion criteria because of lack of randomization or other major methodological flaws. As a result, none of the trials included in their analysis had any data regarding sleep quality or architecture.[65]

Given the voluminous data from uncontrolled trials demonstrating the benefits of chronic NIV during sleep, there clearly are ethical concerns in conducting trials where NIV is withheld or patients are randomized to no therapy or oxygen alone.

While the need for more randomized trials no doubt exists, overcoming these ethical concerns may prove challenging. Designs in which NIV is compared with tracheostomy or those that use subjects who refuse therapy may be inherently flawed because of confounding by such factors as disease severity or patient motivation and compliance. Conclusions drawn from such studies regarding cost, survival, or improvements in sleep or quality of life may, therefore, be inaccurate.

IMPLEMENTATION OF NONINVASIVE VENTILATION IN CHRONIC RESPIRATORY FAILURE

While chronic invasive positive-pressure ventilation (using an endotracheal tube or tracheostomy) has been used to treat all forms of respiratory failure successfully, its prolonged use has several major disadvantages. These include maintenance of the tracheostomy itself, regular suctioning, and need for a highly motivated patient or caregiver. Complications related to invasive positive pressure are also well known and include fistulization, repeated respiratory and soft tissue infections, higher risk of nosocomial infection, tracheomalacia, and significant limitations with speech and swallowing.[66–68]

For these reasons, NIV has become the first choice for chronic ventilation in those patients who can cooperate and protect their airway.[1] Application of NIV can be achieved using almost any modern ventilator and either nasal, oral, or oronasal mask interfaces. NIV is easily applied in the home or inpatient setting and most devices available today are portable. From a health care delivery system standpoint, NIV has a number of advantages over invasive methods of mechanical ventilation. These include lower overall costs, better patient comfort and preference, ease of initiation, the need for fewer care providers, and elimination of tracheostomy-related complications.[69] Patients typically report improvement in sleep quality several days to weeks after implementation of NIV, although this requires becoming acclimated and using it regularly (at least 4 hours per night).[59,61,70–72]

Ventilator options are numerous for NIV and include pressure-limited, volume-limited, and pressure-and-volume–limited models.[73] Options for the mode of ventilation are also equally varied and choice depends largely on patient comfort. In general, though, if larger tidal volumes are needed (10–15 mL/kg), volume-limited ventilators in assist/control mode are required.[74,75] On some home ventilator models, this may be accomplished using the spontaneous/timed or S/T mode, which is equivalent to the spontaneous intermittent mandatory ventilation mode.

Pressure-limited ventilators cycle between two preset levels of positive airway pressure, using either flow or time triggers.[76] Newer ventilators combine aspects of both volume and pressure cycling, but are more expensive. Ventilator selection should be guided by characteristics specific to the patient. Higher inspiratory pressures may be needed in very obese patients, or those with thoracic cage abnormalities, while higher expiratory pressures may be necessary in patients with concomitant obstructive sleep apnea to maintain airway patency during sleep.[18,43] Pressure-cycled ventilators may not provide a high enough inspiratory pressure to ensure an adequate tidal volume in the very obese. Therefore, volume-cycled ventilation may be more appropriate in this setting.[18,43] However, in individuals with neuromuscular disease, pressure-cycled ventilation is usually well tolerated.[18] The major caveat to using pressure-cycled ventilators in this population is that most of these ventilators do not have alarms and therefore should be avoided in patients who are completely dependent on NIV. In general, pressure-cycled ventilators are less expensive, lighter, have a more sensitive trigger, and are considered more comfortable to use than volume-cycled ventilators because patients have control over both the tidal volume and frequency.

Interface selection is critical because poorly fitting masks can limit the effectiveness of therapy and are less likely to be used by the patient. Given the large number of commercially available masks from several manufacturers and availability of custom-molded masks, patients should be able to find a comfortable, tight-sealing mask. Air leaks around the mask, skin irritation, and ulceration are all associated with poor mask fit. From a clinical practice standpoint, availability of dedicated personnel to manage patient-interface issues is critical in improving compliance with NIV and ensuring correct treatment implementation. Attending to oral leaks in patients using nasal masks is particularly important, as these are associated with increased nocturnal arousals, sleep fragmentation, and worsened gas exchange.[58,77] Pressure-cycled ventilation may be useful in patients with significant mask leaks, as it is more likely to ensure adequate delivery of tidal volume than volume-cycled ventilation. This is due to the high airflow these ventilators generate to sustain the prerequisite mask pressure.

Because of leaks in the mask and system, the exhaled volume in patients undergoing nasal ventilation is usually lower than the tidal volume set on the ventilator. Therefore, the delivered tidal volume should be increased until the exhaled volume (measured on the ventilator or with a handheld spirometer) is approximately equal to the desired tidal volume.

Exact guidelines for the titration of NIV have not been clearly established. Nonetheless, treatment goals should aim for improvement in clinical symptoms, along with gas exchange. Correction of hypercapnia should be undertaken with monitoring of the $Paco_2$ via arterial blood gas measurement. Measurements of end-tidal carbon dioxide (CO_2) or transcutaneous CO_2 may not be accurate surrogates of the $Paco_2$ and are associated with significant variance.[78–80] Decreasing the $Paco_2$ by 10 to 15 mm Hg and no less than 40 to 45 mm Hg is a reasonable approach.[81] Adequate oxyhemoglobin saturations of 90% or more may be achieved via improved ventilation alone in some patients. Others may require supplemental oxygen, dictating to some degree the choice in ventilator, as not all home units are capable of delivering oxygen.

INDICATIONS AND CONTRAINDICATIONS FOR NONINVASIVE VENTILATION IN CHRONIC RESPIRATORY FAILURE

Noninvasive ventilation can be used in patients with acute and chronic respiratory failure as long as the patients have good laryngeal competence to prevent aspiration, intact upper airway function, secretions that are not copious, relatively normal mental status, and enough ventilatory reserve to remove the mask periodically throughout the day. General indications for initiation of NIV include clinical symptoms related to nocturnal hypoventilation, along with empiric evidence of respiratory failure.[1,18,43,81] These are summarized in **Box 2** and include daytime hypersomnolence, fatigue, and morning headaches.

The major contraindications to NIV are related to inability of the patient to cooperate or tolerate the interface. Other contraindications are relative and include inability to protect the airway, excessive secretions, mental status changes, development of critical illness, need for continuous ventilatory support, and facial abnormalities that would interfere with adequate mask fit.[1,18,43,81] Contraindications are summarized in **Box 3**. While NIV compared with invasive ventilation has fewer side effects, NIV has specific risks. These include the risk of aspiration, mucus plugging due to the lack of direct access to the airway, facial skin damage or necrosis due to chronic mask use, and aerophagia.

Noninvasive Ventilation in Obesity Hypoventilation Syndrome

Obesity is a worldwide epidemic, affecting more than one third of adults in the United States.[82,83]

Box 2
Indications for noninvasive ventilation in chronic respiratory failure

Daytime symptoms associated with hypercapnia, including:

Fatigue

Dyspnea

Morning headache

And one or more of the following:

Respiratory acidosis during sleep (pH less than 7.3)

Greater than a 10 mm Hg increase in $Paco_2$ during sleep or daytime $Paco_2$ 55 mm Hg or more

Oxyhemoglobin saturations 88% or less for 10% or more of monitoring time or for 5 minutes or more, in spite of supplemental oxygen

Cor pulmonale secondary to hypercapnia unresponsive to conventional medical therapy

Maximal inspiratory pressures less than 60 cm H_2O or vital capacity less than 50% predicted in patients with progressive neuromuscular disorders

---

This rise is most pronounced in the morbidly obese, with body mass indices above 40.[83] Mirroring this alarming trend in obesity, associated disease entities, including obstructive sleep apnea and obesity hypoventilation syndrome, have also increased in prevalence.[84] In fact, approximately 10% of patients with obstructive sleep apnea have concomitant obesity hypoventilation syndrome.

While the natural history of obesity hypoventilation syndrome still remains somewhat unclear, accumulating evidence indicates that this disease is associated with significant morbidity and even early mortality.[85,86] Obesity hypoventilation

---

Box 3
Relative contraindications to NIV therapy

Excessive airway secretions

Inability to protect the upper airway

Impaired cough

History of chronic aspiration

Mental status changes making it difficult to cooperate

Acute facial trauma or anatomic abnormalities

Need for continuous ventilatory support

Development of critical illness

---

syndrome, a diagnosis of exclusion, is commonly defined as persistent daytime hypercapnia ($Paco_2$ >45 mm Hg) in the setting of obesity and without other respiratory disease–causing hypoventilation. Clinical features of obesity hypoventilation syndrome include symptoms of daytime hypercapnia (such as fatigue and morning headache), right-sided heart failure/cor pulmonale, $Paco_2$ of 45 mm Hg or more, hypoxia during wakefulness and sleep (arterial oxygen saturation <90%), a greater than 10 mm Hg increase in the $Paco_2$ during sleep (the primary manifestation), and respiratory acidosis (pH <7.3) during sleep.[87–91] Obesity hypoventilation syndrome can lead to chronic respiratory failure in many affected individuals, requiring support with NIV.[92–95] In these individuals, NIV is an effective therapy that can reverse the daytime hypercapnia and hypoxemia associated with obesity hypoventilation syndrome, can sustain this reverse, and can improve daytime hypersomnolence.[96]

Patients with obesity hypoventilation syndrome may have relatively little excessive daytime somnolence in the setting of significant derangements in arterial blood gas concentration. A recent study by Chouri-Pontarollo and colleagues[97] showed that a traditional subjective measure of excessive daytime somnolence, the Epworth Sleepiness Scale, did not predict the degree of daytime hypercapnia in this population. A more objective behavioral test of hypersomnolence, the Oxford Sleep Resistance test, could discern those with normal $Paco_2$ from those with impaired ventilatory response. This study also showed that subjects with the greatest impairments in CO_2 had the most improvement after NIV in measures of daytime hypersomnolence.[97] Furthermore, the investigators were able to demonstrate improvements with NIV in several sleep parameters, including increased amounts of both REM and delta sleep and fewer microarousals throughout the night.[97]

Underlying differences among obesity hypoventilation syndrome patients regarding the nature of their respiratory dysfunction may account for the observation that continuous positive airway pressure (CPAP) alone suffices for some individuals in correcting the physiologic derangements.[88,98] Bannerjee and colleagues,[99] in their cohort of subjects with obesity hypoventilation syndrome, found that 57% responded to CPAP. The remainder of patients required NIV and as a group had refractory hypoxia, higher body mass indices and more sleep-disordered breathing. Volume ventilation may be necessary in a subset of patients, as they might not be able to maintain upper airway patency without a higher peak inspiratory pressure, which can be provided by volume ventilation.[100,101] Treatment of hypoxic individuals with supplemental oxygen alone is considered inadequate[88,96] and will not correct the hypoventilation. Supplemental oxygen alone may also prolong apneas and can worsen the respiratory acidosis in these patients.

In a recent study of obesity hypoventilation syndrome patients without severe nocturnal desaturation, Piper and colleagues[101] randomized subjects to either CPAP or bilevel ventilation. While both groups had improvements in daytime hypercapnia, the group on bilevel had better subjective sleep quality and vigilance testing.

Patients with suspected obesity hypoventilation syndrome should undergo in-laboratory assessment and titration using NIV. To track achievement of adequate nocturnal ventilation, serial blood gas assessments may be necessary. While a standardized protocol for titration of therapy has yet to be established, proposed algorithms call for elimination of apneas and hypopneas (in those patients with obstructive sleep apnea), correction of hypoxia and hypercapnia using positive pressure, and, if needed, supplemental oxygen in a stepwise fashion.[88] Numerous studies have shown that an inspiratory positive air pressure that is 8 to 10 cm H_2O above the expiratory positive air pressure may be necessary to correct hypoxia and hypercapnia.[95] Given the inability of current auto-adjusting CPAP units to detect hypoventilation and hypoxia, at-home titration using these devices is not recommended.[102] While initiating NIV in these patients, it is important not to rapidly correct the $Paco_2$ to the normal range (no more than 10 mm Hg from baseline), since this may result in posthypercapnic metabolic alkalosis. Due to the extensive monitoring needed, effective titration of NIV may therefore necessitate inpatient admission to either the intensive care unit or to a step-down unit, with an in-dwelling arterial line for frequent arterial blood gas monitoring.

Noninvasive Ventilation in Chronic Obstructive Pulmonary Disease

Patients with COPD report worse sleep quality as compared with the general population.[103] On polysomnographic evaluation, COPD patients have diminished REM sleep and total sleep time and are more prone to nocturnal awakenings and sleep stage changes.[39,104]

From a gas exchange standpoint, routine polysomnography is not recommended in the management of COPD patients with respiratory failure.[105] In normal individuals, daytime oxygenation values predict nocturnal desaturation.[39] However, airflow obstruction is also associated with desaturation during sleep. Thus, daytime oxygen saturation measurements for patients with COPD may not accurately predict nocturnal desaturation.[39,106] Therefore, individuals with COPD in whom long-term oxygen therapy is being considered should undergo nocturnal oximetry to ensure adequate oxygen delivery during sleep.

Obstructive sleep apnea should be considered as a comorbid condition in COPD patients who are obese and have a crowded upper airway, daytime hypersomnolence, or other risk factors. In a subset of patients, these two disorders may overlap.[107] In this clinical scenario, polysomnography should be performed and initiation of CPAP is appropriate.

In COPD patients without obstructive sleep apnea, the chronic use of CPAP or NIV is more controversial. While long-term oxygen therapy has been shown to improve survival in patients with COPD,[108,109] the addition of NIV has not been shown to further augment survival in these patients in several recent meta-analyses and systematic reviews.[110–112] However, it is unclear if the trials included in these analyses and reviews had adequately implemented NIV. An early trial by Strumpf and colleagues[113] did not demonstrate benefits in either gas-exchange variables or in parameters of sleep quality. The investigators failed to find any significant improvement in sleep latency, sleep efficiency, or total sleep time. However, after excluding 7 patients unable to tolerate NIV and 5 dropouts, the investigators only analyzed 7 subjects out of 19 who were eligible, likely rendering the study underpowered. Two other studies using similar patients with COPD (with or without daytime hypercapnia) have demonstrated improvements in total sleep time, decreased sleep latency, increased REM sleep time,[9,14] and improved respiratory and gas exchange variables with NIV. Both trials were performed in COPD patients with hypercapnia, suggesting that this may be the subset of patients who would potentially benefit from NIV. Careful analysis of the underlying data suggested that only those patients who had significant CO_2 retention were actually the subset of patients that appeared to benefit the most from NIV. Unfortunately, this observation has not been borne out by more recent controlled trials. The recently completed Italian multicenter study on COPD[114] compared oxygen therapy alone versus NIV in addition to oxygen. The majority of subjects in this trial were hypercapnic with a mean $Paco_2$ of 54 mm Hg. Although hypercapnia improved in the NIV group, the investigators found no differences in subjective sleep quality, measures of lung function, or rates of hospitalization.

In addition, survival was similar in both groups. Most recently, investigators from the Australian Trial on Non-invasive Ventilation in Chronic Airflow Limitation[115] examined the impact of NIV on several outcomes, including survival and gas exchange. Subjects in this trial were randomized to either oxygen therapy alone or oxygen therapy in conjunction with NIV. The results of this randomized controlled trial that involved long-term follow-up in 144 subjects will, when published, add significantly to the body of evidence concerning the role of NIV in end-stage COPD. While most of the clinical trial data have not shown significant benefits to long-term NIV in patients with COPD, there is some question as to whether or not the patients in the above-mentioned studies had adequately titrated NIV. Indeed, in the systematic review by Kolodziej and colleagues,[110] the studies employing a nonrandomized, crossover design did demonstrate a significant reduction in $Paco_2$, as well as a reduction in work of breathing with NIV in patients with chronic COPD.[116–118] Those nonrandomized studies used higher inspiratory pressures overall, ranging from 20 to 22 cm H_2O, as compared with the randomized clinical trials, in which inspiratory pressures of 10 to 20 cm H_2O were used.[49,110,116–121] Given the concern that the lower inspiratory pressures used in prior randomized clinical trials might have been insufficient, Windisch and colleagues[16] retrospectively examined the effect of NIV in a cohort of COPD subjects with hypercapnic respiratory failure. Those subjects who achieved maximal reduction in $Paco_2$ required a mean inspiratory pressure of 27.7 cm H_2O to decrease the $Paco_2$ (from 53.3 mm Hg to 46.4 mm Hg, $P < .001$). In addition, this amount of ventilatory support augmented lung function, as forced expiratory volume in 1 second increased 140 mL ($P < .001$). This suggests that, to see an effect on mortality, higher inspiratory pressures, targeting reduction in the $Paco_2$, may be needed in future randomized trials.

Given the current clinical trial data available to date, generalized implementation of NIV therapy in all subjects with COPD is still not recommended.[122] While NIV may benefit those COPD patients with concomitant sleep apnea, further randomized clinical trials are needed to determine the precise implementation of NIV, including patient selection criteria and ventilatory settings, in other patients with hypercapnic respiratory failure due to COPD.

SUMMARY

As technology has improved over the last several decades, NIV has become a first-line therapy in the treatment of chronic respiratory failure from a wide array of causes. Given its ease of implementation and better side effect profile, NIV has supplanted both invasive and negative-pressure ventilation in this patient population. A vast number of uncontrolled trials and case series, along with numerous controlled trials, demonstrate the ability of NIV to improve sleep parameters, such as total sleep time and sleep efficiency, as well as the subjective quality of sleep. While NIV serves as a cornerstone of therapy for obesity hypoventilation syndrome, its benefits for patients with COPD are still controversial. Patients can be successfully placed on NIV for the long term with relatively few side effects and improvements in gas exchange, sleep parameters, and daytime symptoms can be realized within days to weeks. However, better-designed studies aimed at elucidating survival benefits, patient selection criteria, and optimal ventilator settings are needed. In addition, future studies employing polysomnography to determine sleep staging, along with subjective and objective measures of daytime sleepiness, would be helpful to more clearly understand the effects of NIV on sleep.

REFERENCES

1. Clinical indications for noninvasive positive pressure ventilation in chronic respiratory failure due to restrictive lung disease, COPD, and nocturnal hypoventilation—a consensus conference report. Chest 1999;116:521–34.
2. British Thoracic Society Standards of Care Committee. Non-invasive ventilation in acute respiratory failure. Thorax 2002;57:192–211.
3. Bach JR. Amyotrophic lateral sclerosis: prolongation of life by noninvasive respiratory AIDS. Chest 2002;122:92–8.
4. Lyall RA, Donaldson N, Fleming T, et al. A prospective study of quality of life in ALS patients treated with noninvasive ventilation. Neurology 2001;57:153–6.
5. Simonds AK, Muntoni F, Heather S, et al. Impact of nasal ventilation on survival in hypercapnic Duchenne muscular dystrophy. Thorax 1998;53:949–52.
6. Annane D, Quera-Salva MA, Lofaso F, et al. Mechanisms underlying effects of nocturnal ventilation on daytime blood gases in neuromuscular diseases. Eur Respir J 1999;13:157–62.
7. Bott J, Carroll MP, Conway JH, et al. Randomised controlled trial of nasal ventilation in acute ventilatory failure due to chronic obstructive airways disease. Lancet 1993;341:1555–7.
8. Brochard L, Mancebo J, Wysocki M, et al. Noninvasive ventilation for acute exacerbations of chronic

obstructive pulmonary disease. N Engl J Med 1995;333:817–22.

9. Elliott MW, Simonds AK, Carroll MP, et al. Domiciliary nocturnal nasal intermittent positive pressure ventilation in hypercapnic respiratory failure due to chronic obstructive lung disease: effects on sleep and quality of life. Thorax 1992; 47:342–8.

10. Gozal D. Nocturnal ventilatory support in patients with cystic fibrosis: comparison with supplemental oxygen. Eur Respir J 1997;10:1999–2003.

11. Kramer N, Meyer TJ, Meharg J, et al. Randomized, prospective trial of noninvasive positive pressure ventilation in acute respiratory failure. Am J Respir Crit Care Med 1995;151:1799–806.

12. Masa Jimenez JF, Sanchez de Cos Escuin J, Disdier Vicente C, et al. Nasal intermittent positive pressure ventilation. Analysis of its withdrawal. Chest 1995;107:382–8.

13. Meduri GU, Cook TR, Turner RE, et al. Noninvasive positive pressure ventilation in status asthmaticus. Chest 1996;110:767–74.

14. Meecham Jones DJ, Paul EA, Jones PW, et al. Nasal pressure support ventilation plus oxygen compared with oxygen therapy alone in hypercapnic COPD. Am J Respir Crit Care Med 1995;152: 538–44.

15. Windisch W, Dreher M, Storre JH, et al. Nocturnal non-invasive positive pressure ventilation: physiological effects on spontaneous breathing. Respir Physiol Neurobiol 2006;150:251–60.

16. Windisch W, Kostic S, Dreher M, et al. Outcome of patients with stable COPD receiving controlled noninvasive positive pressure ventilation aimed at a maximal reduction of $Pa(CO_2)$. Chest 2005;128: 657–62.

17. Gonzalez MM, Parreira VF, Rodenstein DO. Non-invasive ventilation and sleep. Sleep Med Rev 2002; 6:29–44.

18. Perrin C, D'Ambrosio C, White A, et al. Sleep in restrictive and neuromuscular respiratory disorders. Semin Respir Crit Care Med 2005;26:117–30.

19. Becker HF, Piper AJ, Flynn WE, et al. Breathing during sleep in patients with nocturnal desaturation. Am J Respir Crit Care Med 1999;159:112–8.

20. Douglas NJ, White DP, Pickett CK, et al. Respiration during sleep in normal man. Thorax 1982;37:840–4.

21. Douglas NJ, White DP, Weil JV, et al. Hypoxic ventilatory response decreases during sleep in normal men. Am Rev Respir Dis 1982;125:286–9.

22. Douglas NJ, White DP, Weil JV, et al. Hypercapnic ventilatory response in sleeping adults. Am Rev Respir Dis 1982;126:758–62.

23. Krieger J, Turlot JC, Mangin P, et al. Breathing during sleep in normal young and elderly subjects: hypopneas, apneas, and correlated factors. Sleep 1983;6:108–20.

24. Berthon-Jones M, Sullivan CE. Ventilation and arousal responses to hypercapnia in normal sleeping humans. J Appl Physiol 1984;57:59–67.

25. Berthon-Jones M, Sullivan CE. Ventilatory and arousal responses to hypoxia in sleeping humans. Am Rev Respir Dis 1982;125:632–9.

26. Gothe B, Altose MD, Goldman MD, et al. Effect of quiet sleep on resting and CO2-stimulated breathing in humans. J Appl Physiol 1981;50: 724–30.

27. Lopes JM, Tabachnik E, Muller NL, et al. Total airway resistance and respiratory muscle activity during sleep. J Appl Physiol 1983;54:773–7.

28. Tangel DJ, Mezzanotte WS, White DP. Influence of sleep on tensor palatini EMG and upper airway resistance in normal men. J Appl Physiol 1991;70: 2574–81.

29. Wiegand DA, Latz B, Zwillich CW, et al. Upper airway resistance and geniohyoid muscle activity in normal men during wakefulness and sleep. J Appl Physiol 1990;69:1252–61.

30. Hetzel MR, Clark TJ. Comparison of normal and asthmatic circadian rhythms in peak expiratory flow rate. Thorax 1980;35:732–8.

31. Khatri IM, Freis ED. Hemodynamic changes during sleep. J Appl Physiol 1967;22:867–73.

32. Miller JC, Horvath SM. Cardiac output during human sleep. Aviat Space Environ Med 1976;47: 1046–51.

33. Pengelly LD, Alderson AM, Milic-Emili J. Mechanics of the diaphragm. J Appl Physiol 1971;30:797–805.

34. Tabachnik E, Muller NL, Bryan AC, et al. Changes in ventilation and chest wall mechanics during sleep in normal adolescents. J Appl Physiol 1981; 51:557–64.

35. Arnulf I, Similowski T, Salachas F, et al. Sleep disorders and diaphragmatic function in patients with amyotrophic lateral sclerosis. Am J Respir Crit Care Med 1992;161:849–56.

36. Khan Y, Heckmatt JZ. Obstructive apnoeas in Duchenne muscular dystrophy. Thorax 1994;49:157–61.

37. White JE, Drinnan MJ, Smithson AJ, et al. Respiratory muscle activity and oxygenation during sleep in patients with muscle weakness. Eur Respir J 1995;8:807–14.

38. Remmers JE. Effects of sleep on control of breathing. Int Rev Physiol 1981;23:111–47.

39. Fleetham J, West P, Mezon B, et al. Sleep, arousals, and oxygen desaturation in chronic obstructive pulmonary disease. The effect of oxygen therapy. Am Rev Respir Dis 1982;126:429–33.

40. Sawicka EH, Branthwaite MA. Respiration during sleep in kyphoscoliosis. Thorax 1987;42:801–8.

41. Collard P, Dury M, Delguste P, et al. Movement arousals and sleep-related disordered breathing in adults. Am J Respir Crit Care Med 1996;154: 454–9.

42. Hill NS. Noninvasive ventilation for chronic obstructive pulmonary disease. Respir Care 2004; 49:72–87.

43. Mehta S, Hill NS. Noninvasive ventilation. Am J Respir Crit Care Med 2001;163:540–77.

44. Curran FJ, Colbert AP. Ventilator management in Duchenne muscular dystrophy and postpoliomyelitis syndrome: twelve years' experience. Arch Phys Med Rehabil 1989;70:180–5.

45. Garay SM, Turino GM, Goldring RM. Sustained reversal of chronic hypercapnia in patients with alveolar hypoventilation syndromes. Long-term maintenance with noninvasive nocturnal mechanical ventilation. Am J Med 1981;70:269–74.

46. Splaingard ML, Frates RC Jr, Harrison GM, et al. Home positive-pressure ventilation. Twenty years' experience. Chest 1983;84:376–82.

47. Ellis ER, Bye PT, Bruderer JW, et al. Treatment of respiratory failure during sleep in patients with neuromuscular disease. Positive-pressure ventilation through a nose mask. Am Rev Respir Dis 1987; 135:148–52.

48. Schonhofer B, Geibel M, Sonneborn M, et al. Daytime mechanical ventilation in chronic respiratory insufficiency. Eur Respir J 1997;10:2840–6.

49. Diaz O, Begin P, Torrealba B, et al. Effects of noninvasive ventilation on lung hyperinflation in stable hypercapnic COPD. Eur Respir J 2002; 20:1490–8.

50. Nadar S, Prasad N, Taylor RS, et al. Positive pressure ventilation in the management of acute and chronic cardiac failure: a systematic review and meta-analysis. Int J Cardiol 2005;99:171–85.

51. Moran F, Bradley JM, Jones AP, et al. Non-invasive ventilation for cystic fibrosis. Cochrane Database Syst Rev 2007:CD002769.

52. Fauroux B, Boule M, Lofaso F, et al. Chest physiotherapy in cystic fibrosis: improved tolerance with nasal pressure support ventilation. Pediatrics 1999;103:E32.

53. Holland AE, Denehy L, Ntoumenopoulos G, et al. Non-invasive ventilation assists chest physiotherapy in adults with acute exacerbations of cystic fibrosis. Thorax 2003;58:880–4.

54. Kofler A, Carlesi A, Cutrera R, et al. BiPAP versus PEP as chest physiotherapy in patients with cystic fibrosis (abstract). Pediatr Pulmonol 1998;26(S17): 344.

55. Milross MA, Piper AJ, Norman M, et al. Low-flow oxygen and bilevel ventilatory support: effects on ventilation during sleep in cystic fibrosis. Am J Respir Crit Care Med 2001;163:129–34.

56. Placidi G, Cornacchia M, Polese G, et al. Chest physiotherapy with positive airway pressure: a pilot study of short-term effects on sputum clearance in patients with cystic fibrosis and severe airway obstruction. Respir Care 2006;51:1145–53.

57. Young AC, Wilson JW, Kotsimbos TC, et al. Randomised placebo controlled trial of non-invasive ventilation for hypercapnia in cystic fibrosis. Thorax 2008;63:72–7.

58. Teschler H, Stampa J, Ragette R, et al. Effect of mouth leak on effectiveness of nasal bilevel ventilatory assistance and sleep architecture. Eur Respir J 1999;14:1251–7.

59. Barbe F, Quera-Salva MA, de Lattre J, et al. Long-term effects of nasal intermittent positive-pressure ventilation on pulmonary function and sleep architecture in patients with neuromuscular diseases. Chest 1996;110:1179–83.

60. Hill NS, Eveloff SE, Carlisle CC, et al. Efficacy of nocturnal nasal ventilation in patients with restrictive thoracic disease. Am Rev Respir Dis 1992; 145:365–71.

61. Schonhofer B, Kohler D. Effect of non-invasive mechanical ventilation on sleep and nocturnal ventilation in patients with chronic respiratory failure. Thorax 2000;55:308–13.

62. Bach JR, Alba AS, Saporito LR. Intermittent positive pressure ventilation via the mouth as an alternative to tracheostomy for 257 ventilator users. Chest 1993;103:174–82.

63. Cazzolli PA, Oppenheimer EA. Home mechanical ventilation for amyotrophic lateral sclerosis: nasal compared to tracheostomy-intermittent positive pressure ventilation. J Neurol Sci 1996;139(Suppl): 139.

64. Pehrsson K, Olofson J, Larsson S, et al. Quality of life of patients treated by home mechanical ventilation due to restrictive ventilatory disorders. Respir Med 1994;88:21–6.

65. Annane D, Orlikowski D, Chevret S, et al. Nocturnal mechanical ventilation for chronic hypoventilation in patients with neuromuscular and chest wall disorders. Cochrane Database Syst Rev 2007: CD001941.

66. Niederman MS, Ferranti RD, Zeigler A, et al. Respiratory infection complicating long-term tracheostomy. The implication of persistent gram-negative tracheobronchial colonization. Chest 1984;85:39–44.

67. Stauffer JL, Olson DE, Petty TL. Complications and consequences of endotracheal intubation and tracheotomy. A prospective study of 150 critically ill adult patients. Am J Med 1981;70:65–76.

68. Wood DE, Mathisen DJ. Late complications of tracheotomy. Clin Chest Med 1991;12:597–609.

69. Bach JR, Intintola P, Alba AS, et al. The ventilator-assisted individual. Cost analysis of institutionalization vs rehabilitation and in-home management. Chest 1992;101:26–30.

70. Guilleminault C, Philip P, Robinson A. Sleep and neuromuscular disease: bilevel positive airway pressure by nasal mask as a treatment for sleep disordered

breathing in patients with neuromuscular disease. J Neurol Neurosurg Psychiatry 1998;65:225–32.

71. Highcock MP, Morrish E, Jamieson S, et al. An overnight comparison of two ventilators used in the treatment of chronic respiratory failure. Eur Respir J 2002;20:942–5.

72. Piper AJ, Sullivan CE. Effects of long-term nocturnal nasal ventilation on spontaneous breathing during sleep in neuromuscular and chest wall disorders. Eur Respir J 1996;9:1515–22.

73. Drinkwine J, Kacmarek RM. Noninvasive positive pressure ventilation. Equipment and techniques. Respir Care Clin N Am 1996;2:183–94.

74. Leger P, Jennequin J, Gerard M. Home positive pressure ventilation via nasal mask for patients with neuromuscular weakness or restrictive lung or chest-wall disease. Respir Care 1989;34:73–7.

75. Parreira VF, Jounieaux V, Delguste P, et al. Determinants of effective ventilation during nasal intermittent positive pressure ventilation. Eur Respir J 1997;10:1975–82.

76. Strumpf DA, Carlisle CC, Millman RP, et al. An evaluation of the respironics BiPAP bi-level CPAP device for delivery of assisted ventilation. Respir Care 1990;35:415–22.

77. Meyer TJ, Pressman MR, Benditt J, et al. Air leaking through the mouth during nocturnal nasal ventilation: effect on sleep quality. Sleep 1997;20:561–9.

78. Clark JS, Votteri B, Ariagno RL, et al. Noninvasive assessment of blood gases. Am Rev Respir Dis 1992;145:220–32.

79. Hess D. Capnometry and capnography: technical aspects, physiologic aspects, and clinical applications. Respir Care 1990;35:557–76.

80. Sanders MH, Kern NB, Costantino JP, et al. Accuracy of end-tidal and transcutaneous PCO_2 monitoring during sleep. Chest 1994;106:472–83.

81. Claman DM, Piper A, Sanders MH, et al. Nocturnal noninvasive positive pressure ventilatory assistance. Chest 1996;110:1581–8.

82. Flegal KM, Carroll MD, Ogden CL, et al. Prevalence and trends in obesity among US adults, 1999–2000. JAMA 2002;288:1723–7.

83. Sturm R. Increases in morbid obesity in the USA: 2000–2005. Public Health 2007;121:492–6.

84. Bray GA, Bellanger T. Epidemiology, trends, and morbidities of obesity and the metabolic syndrome. Endocrine 2006;29:109–17.

85. Berg G, Delaive K, Manfreda J, et al. The use of health-care resources in obesity-hypoventilation syndrome. Chest 2001;120:377–83.

86. Nowbar S, Burkart KM, Gonzales R, et al. Obesity-associated hypoventilation in hospitalized patients: prevalence, effects, and outcome. Am J Med 2004; 116:1–7.

87. Sleep-related breathing disorders in adults: recommendations for syndrome definition and measurement techniques in clinical research. The report of an American Academy of Sleep Medicine Task Force. Sleep 1999;22:667–89.

88. Berger KI, Ayappa I, Chatr-Amontri B, et al. Obesity hypoventilation syndrome as a spectrum of respiratory disturbances during sleep. Chest 2001;120: 1231–8.

89. Kessler R, Chaouat A, Schinkewitch P, et al. The obesity-hypoventilation syndrome revisited: a prospective study of 34 consecutive cases. Chest 2001;120:369–76.

90. Olson AL, Zwillich C. The obesity hypoventilation syndrome. Am J Med 2005;118:948–56.

91. Rapoport DM, Garay SM, Epstein H, et al. Hypercapnia in the obstructive sleep apnea syndrome. A reevaluation of the "Pickwickian syndrome". Chest 1986;89:627–35.

92. Guo YF, Sforza E, Janssens JP. Respiratory patterns during sleep in obesity-hypoventilation patients treated with nocturnal pressure support: a preliminary report. Chest 2007;131:1090–9.

93. Janssens JP, Derivaz S, Breitenstein E, et al. Changing patterns in long-term noninvasive ventilation: a 7-year prospective study in the Geneva Lake area. Chest 2003;123:67–79.

94. Kessler R, Chaouat A, Weitzenblum E, et al. Pulmonary hypertension in the obstructive sleep apnoea syndrome: prevalence, causes and therapeutic consequences. Eur Respir J 1996;9:787–94.

95. Mokhlesi B, Kryger MH, Grunstein RR. Assessment and management of patients with obesity hypoventilation- syndrome. Proc Am Thorac Soc 2008;5: 218–25.

96. Masa JF, Celli BR, Riesco JA, et al. The obesity hypoventilation syndrome can be treated with noninvasive mechanical ventilation. Chest 2001;119: 1102–27.

97. Chouri-Pontarollo N, Borel JC, Tamisier R, et al. Impaired objective daytime vigilance in obesity-hypoventilation syndrome: impact of noninvasive ventilation. Chest 2007;131:148–55.

98. Sullivan CE, Berthon-Jones M, Issa FG. Remission of severe obesity-hypoventilation syndrome after short-term treatment during sleep with nasal continuous positive airway pressure. Am Rev Respir Dis 1983;128:177–81.

99. Banerjee D, Yee BJ, Piper AJ, et al. Obesity hypoventilation syndrome: hypoxemia during continuous positive airway pressure. Chest 2007;131: 1678–84.

100. de Lucas-Ramos P, de Miguel-Diez J, Santacruz-Siminiani A, et al. Benefits at 1 year of nocturnal intermittent positive pressure ventilation in patients with obesity-hypoventilation syndrome. Respir Med 2004;98:961–7.

101. Piper AJ, Wang D, Yee BJ, et al. Randomised trial of CPAP vs bilevel support in the treatment of obesity

hypoventilation syndrome without severe nocturnal desaturation. Thorax 2008;63(5):395–401.

102. Mokhlesi B, Tulaimat A. Recent advances in obesity hypoventilation syndrome. Chest 2007; 132:1322–36.

103. Breslin E, van der Schans C, Breukink S, et al. Perception of fatigue and quality of life in patients with COPD. Chest 1998;114:958–64.

104. Cormick W, Olson LG, Hensley MJ, et al. Nocturnal hypoxaemia and quality of sleep in patients with chronic obstructive lung disease. Thorax 1986;41: 846–54.

105. Douglas NJ, Flenley DC. Breathing during sleep in patients with obstructive lung disease. Am Rev Respir Dis 1990;141:1055–70.

106. Plywaczewski R, Sliwinski P, Nowinski A, et al. Incidence of nocturnal desaturation while breathing oxygen in COPD patients undergoing long-term oxygen therapy. Chest 2000;117:679–83.

107. Flenley DC. Sleep in chronic obstructive lung disease. Clin Chest Med 1985;6:651–61.

108. Continuous or nocturnal oxygen therapy in hypoxemic chronic obstructive lung disease: a clinical trial. Nocturnal Oxygen Therapy Trial Group. Ann Intern Med 1980;93:391–8.

109. Long term domiciliary oxygen therapy in chronic hypoxic cor pulmonale complicating chronic bronchitis and emphysema. Report of the Medical Research Council Working Party. Lancet 1981;1:681–6.

110. Kolodziej MA, Jensen L, Rowe B, et al. Systematic review of noninvasive positive pressure ventilation in severe stable COPD. Eur Respir J 2007;30: 293–306.

111. Lightowler JV, Wedzicha JA, Elliott MW, et al. Non-invasive positive pressure ventilation to treat respiratory failure resulting from exacerbations of chronic obstructive pulmonary disease: Cochrane systematic review and meta-analysis. BMJ 2003;326:185.

112. Wijkstra PJ, Lacasse Y, Guyatt GH, et al. A meta-analysis of nocturnal noninvasive positive pressure ventilation in patients with stable COPD. Chest 2003;124:337–43.

113. Strumpf DA, Millman RP, Carlisle CC, et al. Nocturnal positive-pressure ventilation via nasal mask in patients with severe chronic obstructive pulmonary disease. Am Rev Respir Dis 1991;144:1234–9.

114. Clini E, Sturani C, Rossi A, et al. The Italian multicentre study on noninvasive ventilation in chronic obstructive pulmonary disease patients. Eur Respir J 2002;20:529–38.

115. O'Donoghue FJ, Catcheside PG, Ellis EE, et al. Sleep hypoventilation in hypercapnic chronic obstructive pulmonary disease: prevalence and associated factors. Eur Respir J 2003;21:977–84.

116. Ambrosino N, Nava S, Bertone P, et al. Physiologic evaluation of pressure support ventilation by nasal mask in patients with stable COPD. Chest 1992; 101:385–91.

117. Krachman SL, Quaranta AJ, Berger TJ, et al. Effects of noninvasive positive pressure ventilation on gas exchange and sleep in COPD patients. Chest 1997;112:623–38.

118. Nava S, Ambrosino N, Rubini F, et al. Effect of nasal pressure support ventilation and external PEEP on diaphragmatic activity in patients with severe stable COPD. Chest 1993;103:143–50.

119. Garrod R, Mikelsons C, Paul EA, et al. Randomized controlled trial of domiciliary noninvasive positive pressure ventilation and physical training in severe chronic obstructive pulmonary disease. Am J Respir Crit Care Med 2000;162:1335–41.

120. Gay PC, Hubmayr RD, Stroetz RW. Efficacy of nocturnal nasal ventilation in stable, severe chronic obstructive pulmonary disease during a 3-month controlled trial. Mayo Clin Proc 1996;71:533–42.

121. Renston JP, DiMarco AF, Supinski GS. Respiratory muscle rest using nasal BiPAP ventilation in patients with stable severe COPD. Chest 1994;105: 1053–60.

122. Global strategy for the diagnosis, management and prevention of COPD, Global Initiative for Chronic Obstructive Lung Disease (GOLD) 2007. Available at: http://www.goldcopd.org. Accessed June 7, 2007.

Sleep in the Intensive Care Unit

Steven Kadiev, MBBCh*, Naeem Ali, MD

KEYWORDS

- Sleep deprivation • Sleep disruption
- Intensive Care Unit (ICU) • Sedation
- Sleep interventions

Sleep is a biologic phenomenon that has been incompletely explained by researchers despite decades of research. The understanding of normal sleep biology has long been informed by the understanding of the pathophysiology of a deficiency of normal sleep. Sleep deprivation (SD) often incapacitates patients and results in significant anxiety and depression. This occurs because normal mechanisms that maintain homeostasis are disrupted for a variety of intrinsic and extrinsic reasons. Although SD is common, it has only recently been suggested that sleep disruption, fragmentation, and deficiency are particularly prevalent in patients cared for in the critical care environment.[1] Unfortunately, the effects of poor sleep quality on the outcomes of critically ill patients are not well understood. This lack of understanding is at least partly related to the lack of normative data on sleep in critical illness. Given the understanding of the importance of sleep fragmentation on stressing the physiology of otherwise healthy adults, it is likely that sleep fragmentation may influence multiple aspects of a critically ill patient's course, response to treatment, and ultimate outcome.

In this chapter, the authors discuss the evidence that: critically ill patients sleep; why SD in this population is deleterious; and the effects of sedation on sleep quality and efficiency. Additionally, the authors comment on a variety of interventions that have been used in the ICU to modify sleep, including pharmacologic and nonpharmacologic methods.

SLEEP PHYSIOLOGY

It is hypothesized that sleep results in restoration of neural substrates that are required for normal cognitive processes.[2] Current evidence that this occurs is indirect or equivocal.[2] Several studies of brain basal metabolism suggest an enhanced synthesis of macromolecules such as nucleic acids and proteins in the brain during sleep. However, data regarding this theory remain scarce, controversial and, importantly for this discussion, are completely lacking in critically ill patients.[3]

Sleep is subdivided into two general states: non-rapid eye movement sleep (NREM) and REM sleep. NREM sleep is further subdivided into four NREM stages.[4] The function of NREM sleep is uncertain, although stages 3 and 4 have been reported to be associated with restorative functions of sleep, namely restoration of alertness and energy.[4] Functional imaging (positron emission tomography, PET) has suggested that there are relative increases in glucose use in the basal forebrain, hypothalamus, ventral striatum, hippocampus and pontine reticular formation during NREM sleep. These are new observations that are in accordance with the view that NREM sleep is important to brain plasticity in homeostatic regulation and mnemonic processing.[5]

Stage REM in healthy adults occurs on average every 90 to 120 minutes and is characterized by a low voltage fast electroencephalogram (EEG) pattern, inactivity of all voluntary muscles except the extraocular muscles, and rapid eye movements.[4] Again, as for NREM sleep, the function of REM sleep is uncertain, however, it may be important for memory consolidation.[6] In fact, Maquet and colleagues[6] using PET and statistical parametric mapping in healthy right-handed volunteers demonstrated that cerebral blood flow is increased to both amygdaloid complexes during

Division of Pulmonary, Allergy, Critical Care and Sleep Medicine, The Ohio State University, 201 DHLRI, 473 West 12th Avenue, Columbus, OH 43210, USA
* Corresponding author.
E-mail address: steven.kadiev@osumc.edu (S. Kadiev).

Sleep Med Clin 3 (2008) 569–580
doi:10.1016/j.jsmc.2008.08.008
1556-407X/08/$ – see front matter. Published by Elsevier Inc.

REM sleep periods. This is relevant as this region is considered important in the acquisition of emotionally influenced memories. These results may provide evidence that certain types of memories are processed during REM sleep. This may be particularly important given the growing knowledge about the prevalence of post-traumatic stress disorder (PTSD) and its relation to sedative use.[7]

LACK OF CLINICAL TOOLS TO MONITOR SLEEPING BEHAVIOR IN CRITICALLY ILL PATIENTS

There is currently no reliable clinical method or scale to assess whether critically ill patients admitted to the ICU sleep. Certainly, subjective observation can allow clinicians to infer that patients sleep. This is, however, inherently limited to the behavioral characteristics of sleep and cannot accurately distinguish between wakefulness (with eyes closed), NREM, and REM stages of sleep. This in sharp comparison to the Richmond Agitation and Sedation Score (RASS), which uses a descriptive numerical scale.[8] The RASS is potentially more accurate than subjective assessments of sleep because with the RASS, alertness and arousability to external stimuli are simultaneously assessed.[8] However, after subjects are deemed to appear to be asleep and are sufficiently unresponsive to stimuli, this scale cannot differentiate between persistent coma and transient sleep.

EEG ASSESSMENT

Despite certain technical issues, there is accumulating evidence that portable monitoring in critically ill ICU patients is feasible and potentially useful. Wright has described their use of continuous EEG monitoring in neurosurgical ICU patients.[9] Although this continuous monitoring provides the benefit of real-time information regarding seizure activity, level of consciousness, and response to therapy, the technique remains fairly impractical because it is labor intensive and the signal is often prone to interference from ICU equipment.[9] However, in certain subjects, it may provide invaluable information and lead to appropriate therapeutic interventions. Crippen described that such computer processed, bedside electroencephalography can provide real-time assessment of brain activity during therapeutic neuromuscular blockade.[10] Sedation and sleep patterns can, therefore, be continuously assessed and inadvertent over-sedation avoided.[10] Technically, electroencephalography is facilitated by the placement of soft, moist contact electrodes across the forehead after skin preparation with

an anti-oil solution. This procedure is quick and easy and does not require sophisticated training.[10]

PORTABLE MONITORING

There are various types of polysomnographic monitoring. Type 1 consists of full overnight polysomnography (PSG), with a minimum of two channels each for EEG, chin electromyogram, electrooculogram, as well as respiratory airflow (with thermistor or pressure-flow transducer), respiratory effort (thoracic and abdominal breathing movements), oximetry, and electrocardiogram or heart rate monitoring. These studies are fully attended by a technologist and are typically conducted in a sleep center.[11] Types 2 to 4 describe portable studies. Type 2 is a portable study with an equal number of physiologic signals and monitored channels as type 1, but can run in the absence of a dedicated technician. Type 3 uses at least four channels, including two channels for respiration and one channel for cardiac monitoring. Type 4 is made up of only one or two channels, typically including oxygen saturation or airflow.[11]

TREATMENT EFFECTS ON SLEEP ARCHITECTURE

There are multiple pharmacologic agents that are in common use in ICU patients that have the potential to disrupt sleep (**Table 1**).[12] For example, sedated, critically ill patients who receive sympathomimetic cardiovascular support may experience sleep disturbances as both vasoactive agents and benzodiazepines can penetrate the blood brain barrier.[12] In such patients D_2-receptor agonism may potentially decrease slow wave and REM sleep, while epinephrine and norepinephrine may decrease REM sleep alone.[12] Amiodarone is another commonly used cardiac medication, which is often prescribed to control and treat atrial fibrillation. Occasionally, it appears to induce nightmares that may have a minor or significant sleep disruptive effect.[13] Patients ventilated and sedated for status asthmaticus may also be at risk of sleep disorders. This is related to the administration of high dose nebulized beta-receptor agonists and high-dose intravenous corticosteroids, the latter reducing both slow wave and REM sleep.[14,15]

Betalactam antibiotics may result in sleep disruption and agitation. This effect, however, may be partially related to increased levels of the inflammatory cytokine, interleukin-6.[16] Quinolones have been associated with insomnia. This adverse effect can be managed with benzodiazepine (BDZ) boluses or alternatively decreasing the quinolone dose.[17] Many antidepressants have sedative effects and therefore may be used to treat

Table 1
Drugs commonly used in the ICU and their effects on sleep architecture

Drug Class or Individual Drug	Sleep Disorder Induced or Reported	Possible Mechanism
Benzodiazepines	↓REM, ↓SWS	Gamma aminobutyric acid type A receptor stimulation
Opioids	↓REM, ↓SWS	μ receptor stimulation
Clonidine	↓REM	α_2 receptor stimulation
Non steroidal anti-inflammatory drugs	↓TST, ↓SE	Prostaglandin synthesis inhibition
Norepinephrine/Epinephrine	Insomnia, ↓REM, ↓SWS	α_1 receptor stimulation
Dopamine	Insomnia, ↓REM, ↓SWS	D_2 receptor stimulation/ α_1 receptor stimulation
β-Blockers	Insomnia, ↓REM, Nightmares	Central nervous system β-blockade by lipophillic agents
Amiodarone	Nightmares	Unknown mechanism
Corticosteroids	Insomnia, ↓REM, ↓SWS	Reduced melatonin secretion
Aminophylline	Insomnia, ↓REM, ↓SWS, ↓TST, ↓SE	Adenosine receptor antagonism
Quinolones	Insomnia	Gamma aminobutyric acid type A receptor inhibition
Tricyclic antidepressants	↓REM	Antimuscarinic activity and α_1 receptor stimulation
Selective serotonin reuptake inhibitors	↓REM, ↓TST, ↓SE	Increased serotonergic activity
Phenytoin	↑Sleep Fragmentation	Inhibition of neuronal calcium influx
Phenobarbital	↓REM	Increased gamma aminobutyric acid type A activity
Carbamazepine	↓REM	Adenosine receptor stimulation and/or serotonergic activity

Abbreviations: REM, rapid eye movement; SWS, slow wave sleep; SE, sleep efficiency; TST, total sleep time.
From Bourne RS, Mills GH. Sleep disruption in critically ill patients—pharmacological considerations. Anaesthesia 2004;59:374; with permission.

insomnia.[18] An important caveat is that they decrease REM sleep and have a minimal effect on slow wave sleep (SWS). This is probably mediated through positive serotonergic effects, especially 5-hydroxytryptamine type 1 A agonism.[18]

Therefore, it is important to understand and recognize that many pharmacologic agents used in the ICU can disrupt normal sleep architecture. It is unclear how these effects could impact short-term outcome, but, given the possibility of potentiating patient stress and adverse patient recall, medication regimens should be reviewed on a daily basis so that such effects are limited.

EVIDENCE THAT CRITICALLY ILL PATIENTS EXPERIENCE SLEEP IN THE ICU

Previous studies have determined that acutely ill patients in the ICU suffer unique sleep disturbances.[19–22] Sleep is fragmented by frequent arousals and awakenings, resulting in decreased or absent SWS and REM stage sleep.[20,21] NREM stage 1 and 2 are increased while total sleep time (TST) is decreased.[20] Additionally, the circadian rhythm of sleep is distorted, with nearly half of the TST occurring during the daytime.[19] As evidence of this, a study analyzing the circadian periodicity of melatonin in critically ill patients revealed significantly deranged biorhythms as compared with healthy control subjects.[23] The irregularity of light stimuli certainly was one factor that likely contributed to this observation, but drug or other treatments that could effect the pineal gland could also play a role. Other factors that have been implicated in possibly disrupting sleep include noise, frequent patient-care activities, medication effects, acute and chronic illness, and dyssynchrony between the patient and the ventilator.[19]

Despite the general acceptance of these changes to normal sleep physiology in critically ill patients, there are many technical issues that make monitoring and objectively assessing sleep physiology difficult. Because the ability to describe sleep is predicated on its accurate physiologic description, these issues impede research in this area. Traditional conditions required for an attended diagnostic polysomnographic recording are impossible to achieve in the ICU setting. Despite this obstacle, several techniques have been used or are currently of potential value for this purpose.

Objective Measures

Polysomnography-electroencephalography
Polysomnography-electroencephalography (PSG-EEG) is performed either in a sleep laboratory or via portable units as described above.[11] Type 1 monitoring is the gold standard for diagnosing sleep disorders and requires that patients be studied in a dedicated sleep laboratory.[11] Although portable studies provide valuable information, collected data is often flawed resulting in high false-negative rates.[24,25]

Bispectral-index
In essence, bispectral-index (BIS) monitoring represents quantitative EEG analysis and has Food and Drug Administration (FDA) approval to measure sedation levels of patients in the operating room and the ICU.[9,26] It has also been used in tracking global cerebral ischemia.[27] The numerical score is complexly derived from statistical processing of the EEG signal. Data input is generated from a 4-lead EEG tracing, and results are compared with a library of known tracings.[9] A numeric score of 0 (electrocerebral silence) to 100 (normal, alert) is subsequently displayed on a bedside computer monitor.[9] Ten subjects undergoing evaluation for obstructive sleep apnea with standard overnight PSG-EEG had concurrent BIS monitoring.[28] Results revealed that mean BIS scores decreased with increasing sleep depth. There was, however, a wide distribution of values at each sleep stage with considerable overlap. Therefore, BIS levels did not reliably correlate with conventionally determined sleep stages. In addition, the response of the BIS was slow and patients could arouse with low BIS values, which then took some time to increase.[28] Turkmen and colleagues[8] evaluated the correlation between BIS monitoring and RASS scores in eleven sedated ICU patients. Data were collected hourly for 8 hours. Significant correlation was noted between the two monitoring systems with mean RASS scores ranging from 0.9 to −1.7 while mean BIS-indices ranged between

65 and 75.[8] As there appears to be conflicting data regarding the BIS-index, its use should probably be limited to investigational research or only as an adjunct in the clinical care of ICU patients.

Actigraph
Use of the actigraph is a one-dimensional method for monitoring sleep.[29] The actigraph is placed either on the wrist or ankle and used to measure patient activity.[30] The device is small, lightweight, and measures gross motor activity and integrates degree and intensity of motion. It contains an accelerometer that is capable of sensing any motion with a minimal resultant force of 0.01 g.[30] Sleep patterns were assessed in an observational study of 68 osteoporotic women via both PSG and actigraphy. Sleep parameters from actigraphy (specifically, proportional integration mode [PIM]) corresponded reasonably well to PSG in this population.[31] Shilo and colleagues[23] used actigraphy to study sleep patterns ICU patients. Disrupted sleep was found in most individuals and this was accompanied by abnormal melatonin secretion. This could therefore be a reasonable and objective method to follow sleep patterns in critically ill patients. The caveat is that paralyzed patients, either via intentional pharmacologic agents or due to underlying pathology, could not be monitored in this way.

Subjective Measures

Patient and nursing assessments
In a surgical ICU population of 104 nonventilated patients, sleep was assessed by both nursing observations and a subjective patient questionnaire (five-item Richards-Campbell Sleep Questionnaire).[32] Results revealed that patients' perceived inadequate sleep while in the ICU, but the nurses' perceptions only partially coincided with those of the patients. Furthermore, patients also tended to overestimate their sleep.[32] Neuromuscular blocking agents (NMBAs) are necessary at times to facilitate mechanical ventilation. Although anxiolytic and sedative medications are routinely administered, patients have reported feeling "buried alive," have recollection of events, and complain of poor sleep while receiving mechanical ventilation and/or NMBAs.[20]

SLEEP DEPRIVATION IS DELETERIOUS TO CRITICALLY ILL PATIENTS

Animal data suggests that severe SD may lead to death.[33] In humans, SD can have significant repercussions although it is rarely so severe and it is unlikely to produce such dramatic consequences. On the other hand, given that SD in sublethal amounts is commonly endured by critically ill patients, it is possible that there are tangible consequences. SD has been shown to decrease immunity, impair cognitive function, increase protein catabolism (via increased metabolic rate), and alter respiratory mechanics.[1,20] These effects, in turn, could negatively impact tolerance to many ICU interventions, weaning from mechanical ventilation, and the avoidance of nosocomial infections.

Immune Function

Sleep deprived-induced immune dysfunction has been associated with neutropenia, lymphopenia, dysfunctional natural-killer cells and polymorphonucleocytes, impaired antigen-specific defenses, and increased mortality.[1,34,35] Shearer and colleagues[36] have shown that total SD over a four-day period results in increased levels of interleukin-6 and soluble tumor necrosis factor-α receptor. Such changes in the immune system have been associated with reactivation of latent viral infections and the development of certain malignancies.[36] Lange and colleagues[37] revealed that healthy subjects who had regular sleep after hepatitis A (HAV) vaccination displayed a nearly twofold higher HAV antibody titer at 4 weeks compared with healthy subjects that were sleep deprived for the first 24 hours after vaccination. Given the multiple other reasons for nosocomial infections, this, in theory, could represent a cofactor in the development of ventilator-associated pneumonia, catheter-related blood stream infections, or poor wound healing in ICU patients. However, a direct relationship between severity of

illness and the degree of immune dysfunction resulting from SD remains to be established.[1]

A substantial proportion of patients admitted to the medical ICU have severe sepsis, with an estimated prevalence of 2.26 cases per 100 hospital discharges.[38] In these cases, patients with localized infection become unable to contain the effects of the pathogen and a generalized systemic response follows. It is unclear why similar patients may clinically respond to standard treatments, while others develop severe sepsis. Clinically, this is characterized by severe vasodilation, abnormal coagulation, organ failure, and possible death.[39] Bacterial products in these septic patients result in activation of inflammatory signaling cascades, which can lead to dysregulation of the innate immune system. Therefore, patients with severe sepsis who become sleep deprived while cared for in the ICU may have augmented immune dysfunction. This may certainly impede recovery and ultimately have a negative impact on ICU outcomes.

Delirium

Delirium in the ICU patient is a common problem and is associated with increased morbidity and mortality, prolonged hospital stay, more diagnostic tests and consultations, and therefore, increased cost of care.[40] The etiology of delirium is usually said to be multifactorial (**Table 2**) with the number of contributors generally being even higher in ICU patients.[41] Importantly, the high prevalence of sleep-wake cycle disruption in ICU

Table 2
Etiology of ICU-associated delirium

Primary brain disease	CVA, malignancy, subdural hematoma, space-occupying lesions, head trauma, seizures
Infections	Brain, chest, urinary, sepsis
Metabolic disorders	Hypoxemia, hypoglycemia, hyperthermia, dehydration, electrolyte imbalances
Medications	Benzodiazepines, morphine, fentanyl, meperidine, propofol
Toxins	
Drug withdrawal	Drugs of abuse, sedation
Sleep deprivation	—
Untreated pain	
Cardiovascular	CHF, myocardial infarction, pulmonary embolus, peripheral vascular disease, gangrene
Gastrointestinal hemorrhage	
Anemia	
Fractures	Hip, pelvis

Abbreviations: CHF, congestive heart failure; CVA, cerebrovascular accident.

patients is now recognized and accepted as an etiologic factor for delirium in this population,[42] although the biologic plausibility remains to be demonstrated. Acute brain dysfunction presenting as delirium can result in impaired short- and long-term cognitive function, behavioral changes, and even psychosis.[1,20,42,43] Hanania and colleagues[42] described the use of melatonin in two postoperative surgical patients. In one individual melatonin was used as prophylaxis against delirium that had occurred after a previous surgery. The second individual developed postoperative sleep-deprived delirium that was refractory to conventional treatment. This resolved after melatonin was instituted. Although they are only case studies, these observations provide some evidence that melatonin may restore the sleep-wake cycle in postoperative patients and this restoration may have an impact on delirium.

This finding is important as the same phenomenon appears to be present in medical ICU patients. Olofsson and colleagues[44] reported that individuals in a medical ICU have disrupted circadian melatonin cycles and they concluded that this probably impacts normal sleep-wake physiology. Possible explanations for this disruption include an abnormal daylight/nightlight relationship, pharmacologic agents used in the ICU, and elevated cortisol levels.[44]

Seizure Threshold

SD is known to facilitate both seizures and interictal epileptiform abnormalities and is therefore often used in the routine diagnostic workup of epileptic patients.[45] Scalise and colleagues[45] studied the effects of SD on cortical excitability in healthy subjects by transcranial magnetic stimulation. Their results suggest that SD modifies the balance between inhibitory and excitatory cortical phenomena, which in turn results in a reduced epileptic threshold. Whether these effects occur in critically ill patients is unknown, however, given this known pathophysiologic relationship, mitigating the potential effects of SD in ICU patients with status epilepticus becomes paramount. How this observation affects other critically ill patients is unknown.

Hyperalgesia

Disturbed sleep is observed in association with acute and chronic pain, and some data suggest that disturbed and shortened sleep enhances pain.[46] Roehrs and colleagues[46] showed that the loss of four hours of sleep (specifically REM sleep) is hyperalgesic on the subsequent day. This is obviously imperative in the ICU patient because there is usually a baseline level of pain and discomfort which could, in theory, be accentuated by SD. It is plausible that the cumulative effects of SD could result in hyperalgesia and, in turn, increased demand for narcotic analgesics. This response could erroneously be interpreted as tolerance, a new pathologic process, or even as narcotic-seeking behaviors. Independent of this, in mechanically-ventilated patients, increased use of medicines that result in sedation has been shown to lead to a longer duration of mechanical ventilation and worse overall recovery.[47]

Ventilatory Consequences

24-hour SD in normal volunteers resulted in a 14% reduction in supine maximal voluntary ventilation (MVV) compared with individuals that had normal sleep.[48,49] Furthermore, supine compared with upright positioning in healthy subjects has been associated with a 10% decrement in MVV. It is therefore conceivable that supine positioning and SD in ICU patients could decrease MVV by approximately 20%.[48] This would obviously influence mechanical ventilation and impact ventilator weaning. Given that ventilatory demands are commonly increased in critically ill patients above normal physiologic values, these changes may have a more dramatic effect than would otherwise be predicted. Possible proposed mechanisms responsible for such sleep-deprived ventilatory insufficiency are respiratory muscle fatigue and decreased neurologic drive.[49-51]

Cardiovascular Consequences

In ambulatory patients, sleep fragmentation can result in elevations of arterial blood pressure, elevations of urinary and serum catecholamines, arrhythmias, progression of cardiac failure, and even death.[52] SD might cause similar abnormalities in critically ill patients, although direct evidence is lacking.[52] However, given the frequency with which the cardiovascular system is monitored in critically ill patients and the fact that this monitoring drives treatment decisions or the assessment of physiologic recovery, confounding the observations of these parameters could lead to unnecessary therapy.

DOES SEDATION EQUAL SLEEP?

Critically ill patients are often given sedatives to increase patient comfort, decrease anxiety and agitation, promote amnesia, and provide tolerance to life support. Their use, however, may prolong both the duration of mechanical ventilation by 2.5 days and ICU stay by 3.5 days.[52-54] Despite the behavioral similarity to physiologic sleep (sedentary with diminished responsiveness to external stimuli), there is little data to answer the question of whether sedative-induced sleep is restorative.

Helping to understand this complex issue, Hardin and colleagues[20] studied 18 patients with respiratory failure requiring mechanical ventilation. Patients received lorazepam and morphine via intermittent bolus doses (intermittent sedation [IS]), continuous sedation (CS), and CS with NMBAs. As expected all patients displayed abnormal sleep-wake cycles with erratic progression through the sleep stages. Overall mean TST approximated normal values. Amongst the three sedation strategies, TST was increased in patients receiving CS, but greater than 50% of sleep occurred during the daytime period. This increase in TST appeared to come at the cost of disruption of nighttime sleep and alteration in normal circadian rhythm. It is uncertain whether these costs are greater than the prevention of sleep deprivation.[20] REM sleep was severely reduced in all of the studied groups, with only patients in the IS group having any consistently detectable sleep time in this category. Only 50% of those on continuous sedatives manifest REM sleep whereas subjects with NMBAs were unable to demonstrate muscle tone changes to even make detection possible. Alarmingly, patients receiving NMBAs spent 22% of the sleep period awake, highlighting the difficulty with using physical observation as the primary way to characterize sleep and comfort.[20]

In a separate descriptive series of 20 critically ill medical-surgical ICU patients that required intubation and mechanical ventilation,[21] PSG was performed in all patients while sedated with various opiates and BDZs. None of the subjects exhibited normal sleep patterns by PSG. Sleep could only be characterized into three groups: (1) disrupted sleep: abnormal circadian rhythm, increased stage 1 NREM sleep and reduced REM sleep, severe

sleep fragmentation; (2) atypical sleep: transitions from stage 1 NREM to slow wave sleep with a virtual absence of stage 2 NREM and reduced stage REM sleep; (3) coma: characterized by > 50% delta or theta EEG activity.[21] Higher doses of sedative medications resulted in increased atypical sleep and EEG patterns more suggestive of encephalopathy and coma. However, the authors indicate that this observation may have been confounded by the presence of concomitant renal failure, which was present in a number of study subjects. Taken together these studies emphasize that increased sedation results in disrupted sleep architecture, which may impede the normal restorative functions of sleep. Given the recent data about the deleterious consequences of excessive BDZ use in critically ill patients, it is possible that sleep disruption is a mediator of these effects.

SLEEP INTERVENTIONS IN THE ICU

With critically ill patients, restoring normal sleep architecture should be the goal. However, given the current understanding of sleep in critically ill patients, it is unclear what the most appropriate therapeutic target should be. Should research focus on consolidating sleep or merely extending TST in a 24-hour interval? Separately, should researchers worry that induction of Stage 3 or 4 sleep may in fact be abnormal based on the age of the patient in question and the potential for prolonging immobilization? Despite these concerns, several interventions have been proposed and studied in critically ill patients. These various interventions are summarized in **Table 3**.

Pharmacologic

Medications
As SD is prevalent in ICU patients, it is likely important to facilitate physiologic sleep to prevent possible deleterious effects associated with this

---

Table 3
Sleep interventions for critically ill ICU patients

Pharmacologic	Nonpharmacologic
Medications – adjuncts	Environmental
Melatonin	Noise abatement
Dexmedetomidine	Light abatement
Minimizing sleep inhibitory medications	Ensure uninterrupted time for adequate sleep
Symptom targeted sedation	Ventilator modes – ensure synchrony
Effective analgesia	Limit nocturnal patient care activities
Sedation holidays	Promote patient orientation
	Relaxation techniques

deficiency state.[19–21] Non-benzodiazepine agents such zolpidem and zopiclone interact with specific gamma aminobutyric acid (GABA) receptor sub-units in contrast to BDZs. It is thought that as a result of this specificity, zolpidem and zopiclone do not suppress SWS, whereas BDZs do.[1] Additionally, these agents suppress REM sleep less than BDZs and may therefore be more optimal in promoting sleep.[1,55] This data was collected from healthy male subjects so one could infer that similar effects could occur in critically ill ICU patients.

BDZs, usually in combination with opioids, are the most commonly prescribed agents used for sedation and anxiolysis in mechanically-ventilated patients in the United States. In healthy subjects, it has been shown that BDZs increase TST, but more importantly, they decrease SWS and REM sleep.[1,56,57] Furthermore, tolerance to BDZs occurs within a few days often resulting in escalating doses. Unfortunately, paradoxical effects such as hallucinations, insomnia, and agitation can occur.[1] PSG was performed pre- and post-operatively in ten women undergoing benign gynecologic surgery. They were randomized to either an opioid or local anesthetic epidural. Results revealed that SWS and REM sleep were significantly lower in the opioid group.[12,58] Therefore, physicians should be cognizant that BDZs and opioids disrupt normal sleep architecture and may impede the restorative functions of sleep.[1]

Shilo and colleagues[59] performed a small double-blind placebo-controlled trial of patients with chronic obstructive pulmonary disease who required ICU admission due to respiratory failure. Sleep was defined by observation and wrist actigraphy. Those who received nightly scheduled controlled-release melatonin had improved sleep duration and quality.[59] Analysis of polysomnographic EEG tracings shows that dexmedetomidine produces a state closely resembling physiologic stage two NREM sleep in humans, which gives further support to earlier experimental evidence for activation of normal NREM sleep-promoting pathways by this sedative agent.[60]

Haloperidol is sometimes used to decrease agitation in ICU patients, and it has been reported to cause sleep disturbances in 4% of patients receiving antipsychotic therapy.[61] Newer, atypical antipsychotics such as risperidone appear to increase slow wave sleep compared with haloperidol, probably due to 5-hydroxytryptamine type 2 antagonist activity and therefore, could be deemed more appropriate in this population.[62]

Agents disrupting sleep
Alcohol, illicit drugs (eg, cocaine) or prescription medications (**Table 1**) can all result in disrupted sleep.[12,63] These illicit or prescription drugs can often be present in critically ill patients through intentional or prescribed ingestion. Awareness of these effects in patients presenting with these medications and awareness of their withdrawal on sleep quality are important to appropriately react to a change in a patient's condition. Therefore, pharmacologic agents used in the ICU should be used judiciously and discontinued when no longer required. Special attention is required for those individuals admitted with alcohol or illicit drug intoxication. These patients often require BDZs, which may further compound their SD.[1]

Nonpharmacologic

Environmental
Noise reduction Numerous studies have examined ICU noise levels, and all have concluded that they exceed Environmental Protection Agency recommendations for hospitals, which are less than 45 decibels (dB) during the daytime and less than 35 dB at night.[19] Because the dB scale is logarithmic, a sound increase of 10 dB is actually perceived as twice as loud.[64] Bursts of sound are known to result in arousal from sleep. The threshold necessary for arousal depends on sleep stage, age of the patient, and habituation to a particular environment.[64] Zeplin and colleagues[65] showed that sound peaks over 70 dB resulted in arousals in both men and women between the ages 52 and 57 in all stages of sleep, and the older the individual, the lower the threshold necessary for arousal.

Gabor and colleagues[19] studied the effect of reducing noise in six healthy volunteers while they slept in an ICU. The average level of noise was 51 dB in an open ICU and 43 dB in an isolated single room (peak levels were 65 and 54 dB respectively). TST was greater in the isolated room than in the open ICU room by approximately 80 minutes (9.5 versus 8.2 hours), although the number of arousals and awakenings were virtually identical in the two settings.[19] Wallace and colleagues[66] found that use of earplugs increased REM sleep and decreased REM latency, although the number of awakenings was not affected. By limiting ICU noise, it is possible that one could increase both TST and REM sleep, possibly facilitating improved sleep architecture.

Light abatement It has been proposed that light exposure, the primary zeitgeber responsible for setting the circadian clock, can also affect the sleep pattern of ICU patients.[22] However, a survey of patients who survived their ICU admission revealed that light was not as disruptive to their sleep as were noise and patient care activities.[67] As a reference, general office room lighting ranges between 320 to 500 lux.[68] In comparison, nocturnal light levels in certain ICUs, were variable, with mean maximum levels ranging between less than 5 lux to more than 1400 lux.[64,69] Light levels as low as 100 to 500 lux have been found to affect nocturnal melatonin secretion, and 300 to 500 lux may have an affect on the human circadian pacemaker.[70] Therefore, the importance of light as a disruptive factor for a patient's sleep and circadian physiology may vary depending on the light level in each ICU. It has been suggested that light abatement performed between 11 PM and 5 AM is associated with reduced sleep disturbances.[71]

Ventilator modes

Mechanically-ventilated patients experience considerable sleep disruption, with as many as 20–63 arousals and awakenings per hour.[19,21,52] Patient ventilator discordance is known to cause this sleep disruption for a variety of reasons including patient comfort and altered ventilation.[72] To determine whether the type of ventilator support affected the amount of sleep disruption, Parthasarathy and Tobin performed PSG on 11 critically ill patients who required mechanical ventilation with either pressure support (PS) or assist-control ventilation (ACV).[73] Compared with ACV, PS resulted in more sleep fragmentation as measured by total arousals and awakenings.[73] The proposed physiologic mechanism responsible for PS-induced arousals is central sleep apneas that arose during this form of mechanical ventilation.[74] Proportional assist ventilation (PAV) is a form of synchronized partial ventilatory assistance where the ventilator generates pressure in proportion to the patient's instantaneous effort, which theoretically could improve patient–ventilator interactions.[75] Bosma and colleagues[72] studied 13 patients undergoing ventilator-weaning in a medical–surgical ICU. They demonstrated that PAV was more efficacious than PS ventilation in matching ventilatory requirements, and resulted in fewer patient–ventilator asynchronies and better quality of sleep during the weaning period.

Patient care activities

Performing routine nocturnal ICU activities such as vital sign assessment, attending to patient hygiene, medication administration, and diagnostic testing results in sleep disruption and may culminate in various deleterious effects. In many observational studies, patient care activities have resulted in significant sleep disruptions. These disruptions have been shown to be minimized by using continuous monitoring (eg, arterial lines and pulse oximetry) instead of manual blood pressure

cuffs with intermittent checks and by limiting invasive procedures and disruptive tests (blood draws, radiography and other testing) to daytime hours.[1]

Relaxation techniques

Richards studied a cohort of critically ill men and found that a daily six-minute back massage resulted in longer TST.[76] Williamson investigated the effects of ocean sounds (white noise) on the nocturnal sleep patterns of postoperative coronary artery bypass graft patients after transfer from an ICU.[77] Outcomes were subjective, recorded with a standard sleep questionnaire. Their results suggested that this simple intervention improved subjective sleep quality.

SUMMARY

It is well established that SD is prevalent in the ICU population.[19–22] It is often multifactorial and related to both the physical ICU environment and to instituted medical care. It is of concern that numerous deleterious effects, such as immune dysfunction and delirium, can ensue after such deprivation.[1,42] The ICU team should therefore adopt an approach that limits sleep disruption. The approach should consist of limiting medications that interfere with normal sleep architecture, providing appropriate pharmacologic adjuncts, and, at a minimum, creating a nocturnal environment that is conducive to sleep. Currently, a number of medications are available to treat sleep disorders, but evidence of efficacy specifically in ICU patients is limited.[12] Further investigation of the benefit of exogenous melatonin, atypical antipsychotics and non-benzodiazepine GABA agents in the resolution of sleep problems in ICU patients is indicated.

REFERENCES

1. Friese RS. Sleep and recovery from critical illness and injury: a review of theory, current practice, and future directions. Crit Care Med 2008;36:697–705.
2. Frank MG. The mystery of sleep function: current perspectives and future directions. Rev Neurosci 2006;17:375–92.
3. Maquet P. Sleep function(s) and cerebral metabolism. Behav Brain Res 1995;69:75–83.
4. Iber C, Ancoli-Israel S, Chesson A, et al. The AASM manual for the scoring of sleep and associated events: rules, terminology, and technical specification. 1st edition. Westchester (Illinois): American Academy of Sleep Medicine; 2007.
5. Nofzinger EA, Buysse DJ, Miewald JM, et al. Human regional cerebral glucose metabolism during non-rapid eye movement sleep in relation to waking. Brain 2002;125:1105–15.

6. Maquet P, Peters J, Aerts J. Functional neuroanatomy of human rapid-eye-movement sleep and dreaming. Nature 1996;383:163–6.

7. Kress JP, Gehlbach B, Lacy M, et al. The long-term psychological effects of daily sedative interruption on critically ill patients. Am J Respir Crit Care Med 2003;168:1457–61.

8. Turkmen A, Altan A, Turgut N, et al. The correlation between the Richmond agitation-sedation scale and bispectral index during dexmedetomidine sedation. Eur J Anaesthesiol 2006;23:300–4.

9. Wright WL. Multimodal monitoring in the ICU: when could it be useful? J Neurol Sci 2007;261:10–5.

10. Crippen D. Role of bedside electroencephalography in the adult intensive care unit during therapeutic neuromuscular blockade. Crit Care 1997;1:15–24.

11. Ahmed M, Patel NP, Rosen I. Portable monitors in the diagnosis of obstructive sleep apnea. Chest 2007;132:1672–7.

12. Bourne RS, Mills GH. Sleep disruption in critically ill patients–pharmacological considerations. Anaesthesia 2004;59:374–84.

13. Reiffel JA. Intravenous Amiodarone in the Management of Atrial Fibrillation. J Cardiovasc Pharmacol Ther 1999;4:199–204.

14. Turner R, Elson E. Sleep disorders. Steroids cause sleep disturbance. BMJ 1993;306:1118–21.

15. Klein-Gitelman MS, Pachman LM. Intravenous corticosteroids: adverse reactions are more variable than expected in children. J Rheumatol 1998;25:1995–2002.

16. Spath-Schwalbe E, Hansen K, Schmidt F, et al. Acute effects of recombinant human interleukin-6 on endocrine and central nervous sleep functions in healthy men. J Clin Endocrinol Metab 1998;83:1573–9.

17. Unseld E, Ziegler G, Gemeinhardt A, et al. Possible interaction of fluoroquinolones with the benzodiazepine-GABAA-receptor complex. Br J Clin Pharmacol 1990;30:63–70.

18. Gillin JC, Jernajczyk W, Valladares-Neto DC, et al. Inhibition of REM sleep by ipsapirone, a 5HT1A agonist, in normal volunteers. Psychopharmacology 1994;116:433–6.

19. Gabor JY, Cooper AB, Crombach SA, et al. Contribution of the intensive care unit environment to sleep disruption in mechanically ventilated patients and healthy subjects. Am J Respir Crit Care Med 2003;167:708–15.

20. Hardin KA, Seyal M, Stewart T, et al. Sleep in critically ill chemically paralyzed patients requiring mechanical ventilation. Chest 2006;129:1468–77.

21. Cooper AB, Thornley KS, Young GB, et al. Sleep in critically ill patients requiring mechanical ventilation. Chest 2000;117:809–18.

22. Weinhouse GL, Schwab RJ. Sleep in the critically ill patient. Sleep 2006;29:707–16.

23. Shilo L, Dagan Y, Smorjik Y, et al. Patients in the intensive care unit suffer from severe lack of sleep associated with loss of normal melatonin secretion pattern. Am J Med Sci 1999;317:278–81.

24. Chesson AL Jr, Berry RB, Pack A. Practice parameters for the use of portable monitoring devices in the investigation of suspected obstructive sleep apnea in adults. Sleep 2003;26:907–13.

25. Flemons WW, Littner MR, Rowley JA, et al. Home diagnosis of sleep apnea: a systematic review of the literature: an evidence review cosponsored by the american academy of sleep medicine, the american college of chest physicians, and the american thoracic society. Chest 2003;124:1543–79.

26. Nasraway SS Jr, Wu EC, Kelleher RM, et al. How reliable is the Bispectral Index in critically ill patients? A prospective, comparative, single-blinded observer study. Crit Care Med 2002;30:1483–7.

27. Geocadin RG. A novel quantitative EEG injury measure of global cerebral ischemia. Clin Neurophysiol 2000;111:1779–87.

28. Nieuwenhuijs D, Coleman EL, Douglas NJ, et al. Bispectral index values and spectral edge frequency at different stages of physiologic sleep. Anesth Analg 2002;94:125–9.

29. Ancoli-Israel S, Cole R, Alessi C, et al. The role of actigraphy in the study of sleep and circadian rhythms. Sleep 2003;26:342–92.

30. Grap MJ, Borchers CT, Munro CL, et al. Actigraphy in the Critically Ill: Correlation With Activity, Agitation, and Sedation. Am J Crit Care 2005;14:52–60.

31. Blackwell T, Redline S, Ancoli-Israel S, et al. Comparison of sleep parameters from actigraphy and polysomnography in older women: the SOF study. Sleep 2008;31:283–91.

32. Nicolas A, Aizpitarte E, Iruarrizaga A, et al. Perception of night-time sleep by surgical patients in an intensive care unit. Nurs Crit Care 2008;13:25–33.

33. Rechtschaffen A, Gilliland MA, Bergmann BM, et al. Physiological correlates of prolonged sleep deprivation in rats. Science 1983;221:182–4.

34. Irwin MR, Wang M, Campomayor CO, et al. Sleep deprivation and activation of morning levels of cellular and genomic markers of inflammation. Arch Intern Med 2006;166:1756–62.

35. Zager A, Andersen ML, Ruiz FS, et al. Effects of acute and chronic sleep loss on immune modulation of rats. Am J Physiol Regul Integr Comp Physiol 2007;293:R504–9.

36. Shearer WT, Reuben JM, Mullington JM, et al. Soluble TNF-alpha receptor 1 and IL-6 plasma levels in humans subjected to the sleep deprivation model

of spaceflight. J Allergy Clin Immunol 2001;107: 165–70.

37. Lange T, Perras B, Fehm HL, et al. Sleep enhances the human antibody response to hepatitis A vaccination. Psychosom Med 2003;65:831–5.

38. Angus DC, Linde-Zwirble WT, Lidicker J, et al. Epidemiology of severe sepsis in the United States: analysis of incidence, outcome, and associated costs of care. Crit Care Med 2001;29:1303–10.

39. Daubeuf B, Mathison J, Spiller S, et al. TLR4/MD-2 monoclonal antibody therapy affords protection in experimental models of septic shock. J Immunol 2007;179:6107–14.

40. Silverstein JH. Risk factors and impact of postoperative delirium in elderly surgical patients. Anesthesiology 1999;91:A13.

41. George J, Bleasdale S, Singleton SJ. Causes and prognosis of delirium in elderly patients admitted to a district general hospital. Age Ageing 1997; 26:423–7.

42. Hanania M, Kitain E. Melatonin for treatment and prevention of postoperative delirium. Anesth Analg 2002;94:338–9.

43. Lipowski ZJ. Delirium (acute confusional states). JAMA 1987;258:1789–92.

44. Olofsson K, Alling C, Lundberg D, et al. Abolished circadian rhythm of melatonin secretion in sedated and artificially ventilated intensive care patients. Acta Anaesthesiol Scand 2004;48:679–84.

45. Scalise A, Desiato MT, Gigli GL, et al. Increasing cortical excitability: a possible explanation for the proconvulsant role of sleep deprivation. Sleep 2006; 29:1595–8.

46. Roehrs T, Hyde M, Blaisdell B, et al. Sleep loss and REM sleep loss are hyperalgesic. Sleep 2006; 29:145–51.

47. Pandharipande P, Shintani A, Peterson J, et al. Lorazepam is an independent risk factor for transitioning to delirium in intensive care unit patients. Anesthesiology 2006;104:21–6.

48. Keeling WF, Martin BJ. Supine position and sleep loss each reduce prolonged maximal voluntary ventilation. Respiration 1988;54:119–26.

49. Chen HI, Tang YR. Sleep loss impairs inspiratory muscle endurance. Am Rev Respir Dis 1989;140: 907–9.

50. Phillips B. Sleep, sleep loss, and breathing. South Med J 1985;78:1483–6.

51. Vassilakopoulos T, Zakynthinos S, Roussos C. Respiratory muscles and weaning failure. Eur Respir J 1996;9:2383–400.

52. Parthasarathy S, Tobin MJ. Sleep in the intensive care unit. Intensive Care Med 2004;30:197–206.

53. Treggiari-Venzi M, Borgeat A, Fuchs-Buder T, et al. Overnight sedation with midazolam or

propofol in the ICU: effects on sleep quality, anxiety and depression. Intensive Care Med 1996;22: 1186–90.

54. Kress JP, Pohlman AS, O'Connor MF, et al. Daily interruption of sedative infusions in critically ill patients undergoing mechanical ventilation. N Engl J Med 2000;342:1471–7.

55. Merlotti L, Roehrs T, Koshorek G, et al. The dose effects of zolpidem on the sleep of healthy normals. J Clin Psychopharmacol 1989;9:9–14.

56. Achermann P, Borbely AA. Dynamics of EEG slow wave activity during physiological sleep and after administration of benzodiazepine hypnotics. Human Neurobiology 1987;6:203–10.

57. Borbely AA, Mattmann P, Loepfe M, et al. Effect of benzodiazepine hypnotics on all-night sleep EEG spectra. Hum Neurobiol 1985;4:189–94.

58. Cronin AJ, Keifer JC, Davies MF, et al. Postoperative sleep disturbance: influences of opioids and pain in humans. Sleep 2001;24:39–44.

59. Shilo L, Dagan Y, Smorjik Y, et al. Effect of melatonin on sleep quality of COPD intensive care patients: a pilot study. Chronobiol Int 2000;17:71–6.

60. Huupponen E, Maksimow A, Lapinlampi P, et al. Electroencephalogram spindle activity during dexmedetomidine sedation and physiological sleep. Acta Anaesthesiol Scand 2008;52:289–94.

61. Heck AH, Haffmans PM, de Groot IW, et al. Risperidone versus haloperidol in psychotic patients with disturbing neuroleptic-induced extrapyramidal symptoms: a double-blind, multi-center trial. Schizophr Res 2000;46:97–105.

62. Hidehisa Y, Shigeru M, Shigeto Y, et al. Effect of risperidone on sleep in schizophrenia: a comparison with haloperidol. Psychiatry Res 2002;109: 137–42.

63. Nagel CL, Markie MB, Richards KC, et al. Sleep promotion in hospitalized elders. Medsurg Nurs 2003; 12:279–89.

64. Meyer TJ, Eveloff SE, Bauer MS, et al. Adverse environmental conditions in the respiratory and medical ICU settings. Chest 1994;105:1211–6.

65. Zepelin H, McDonald CS, Zammit GK. Effects of age on auditory awakening thresholds. J Gerontol 1984; 39:294–300.

66. Wallace CJ, Robins J, Alvord LS, et al. The effect of earplugs on sleep measures during exposure to simulated intensive care unit noise. Am J Crit Care 1999;8:210–9.

67. Freedman NS, Kotzer N, Schwab RJ. Patient perception of sleep quality and etiology of sleep disruption in the intensive care unit. Am J Respir Crit Care Med 1999;159:1155–62.

68. Durak A, Camgoz Olgunturk N, Yener C, et al. Impact of lighting arrangements and illuminances on

different impressions of a room. Building and Environment 2007;42:3476–82.

69. Walder B, Francioli D, Meyer JJ, et al. Effects of guidelines implementation in a surgical intensive care unit to control nighttime light and noise levels. Crit Care Med 2000;28:2242–7.

70. Boivin DB, Duffy JF, Kronauer RE, et al. Dose-response relationships for resetting of human circadian clock by light. Nature 1996;379:540–2.

71. Szokol JW, Vender JS. Anxiety, delirium, and pain in the intensive care unit. Crit Care Clin 2001;17:821–42.

72. Bosma K, Ferreyra G, Ambrogio C, et al. Patient-ventilator interaction and sleep in mechanically versus proportional assist ventilation. Crit Care Med 2007;35:1048–54.

73. Parthasarathy S, Tobin MJ. Effect of ventilator mode on sleep quality in critically ill patients. Am J Respir Crit Care Med 2002;166:1423–9.

74. Cabello B, Parthasarathy S, Mancebo J. Mechanical ventilation: let us minimize sleep disturbances. Curr Opin Crit Care 2007;13:20–6.

75. Ambrosino N, Rossi A. Proportional assist ventilation (PAV): a significant advance or a futile struggle between logic and practice? Thorax 2002;57:272–6.

76. Richards KC. Effect of a back massage and relaxation intervention on sleep in critically ill patients. Am J Crit Care 1998;7:288–99.

77. Williamson JW. The effects of ocean sounds on sleep after coronary artery bypass graft surgery. Am J Crit Care 1992;1:91–7.

Management of Insomnia in Patients with Chronic Pulmonary Disease

James D. Geyer, MD[a,b,]*, Megan E. Ruiter, BS[b],
Kenneth L. Lichstein, PhD[b]

KEYWORDS

• Insomnia • Pulmonary disease

Considerable research has been done to better understand the effects of sleep on obstructive lung diseases, such as chronic obstructive pulmonary disease (COPD). Improved monitoring techniques have shown that sleep may have deleterious effects on oxygenation during sleep. Research involving COPD and sleep has primarily involved breathing and oxygenation, with only scant attention paid to insomnia and other sleep disorders.

Insomnia is a common problem in the chronically ill but has been studied in much less detail than have the sleep-related breathing disorders. Insomnia is in itself not a diagnosis but a category of illness. Sleep onset insomnia and sleep maintenance insomnia are the two most common subcategories of insomnia, both of which can be seen in patients with COPD. Not only does insomnia complicate COPD, but the treatments for insomnia can complicate the management of COPD. The overall impact of insomnia on COPD is only just beginning to be appreciated.

OBSTRUCTIVE LUNG DISEASES
Clinical Epidemiology

Chronic obstructive pulmonary disorder

COPD is one of the most rapidly growing health problems in the United States and ranks as the fourth most common killer.[1] Patients with COPD must also endure the expected sleep-related increase in airway resistance, decreased intercostal muscle activity, and fall in forced residual capacity.[2] Obstructive sleep apnea (OSA) and COPD often exist in the same patient in what is termed overlap syndrome.

Asthma and other obstructive lung diseases

Asthma affects 14 to 15 million people in the United States and is the most common chronic disease in childhood.[3] In a large study of nocturnal symptoms in 7729 asthmatics in the United Kingdom, 74% reported awakening at least once per night and 64% awakened at least three times per night.[4] Patients with insomnia often underestimated the severity of their asthma and were more prone to having allergies; and no particular asthma drug was associated with a lessening of the reported nocturnal symptoms.[4] Serial measurements of peak expiratory airflow have shown that airflow obstruction in asthmatic patients peaks between 3:00 and 4:00 AM.[5]

A more extreme but much less common form of airway disease is cystic fibrosis (CF). It is the most common life-shortening autosomal recessive disorder in the Caucasian population[6] and affects approximately 30,000 persons in the United States. The resulting bronchiectasis, COPD, and chronic recurrent infection account for over 90% of fatalities.

OBSTRUCTIVE SLEEP APNEA

Although OSA is not a chronic pulmonary disorder but a chronic sleep-related breathing disorder,

[a] Alabama Neurology and Sleep Medicine, 100 Rice Mine Road Loop, Suite 301, Tuscaloosa, AL 35406, USA
[b] Department of Psychology, The University of Alabama, Box 870348, Tuscaloosa, AL 35487, USA
* Corresponding author.
E-mail address: JGeyer@nctpc.com (J.D. Geyer).

Sleep Med Clin 3 (2008) 581–588
doi:10.1016/j.jsmc.2008.08.011

OSA is one of the most common disorders of breathing. OSA is increasingly recognized by primary care physicians and specialists; and with the epidemic of obesity, the population is increasingly at risk. OSA is common and, therefore, commonly present in patients with other conditions. Overlap syndrome is a term that has been used to describe the coexistence of OSA and COPD. OSA, however, overlaps with a number of other conditions. Though common, the inter-relationship between insomnia and OSA is rarely recognized, inefficiently treated, and often ignored.

Disease Impact on Sleep

Chronic obstructive pulmonary disease

COPD impacts sleep in several different ways. The impairment in oxygenation associated with COPD can increase the adverse consequences of obstructive or central sleep apnea, resulting in more serious oxygen desaturations. Patients with COPD also tend to have more fragmented sleep. Both sleep maintenance and sleep onset insomnia may complicate the COPD, either by the impact of poor sleep or the use of certain medications. Insomnia may arise as a consequence of the COPD, with sleep fragmentation being the most common form. In addition to sleep fragmentation related to abnormal breathing, the chronic negative reinforcement related to the sleep fragmentation can result in sleep-onset insomnia. The various forms of insomnia may, however, be unrelated to the COPD but complicate its management.

Asthma and other obstructive lung diseases

Polysomnographic studies have demonstrated decreased sleep efficiency, increased arousals and awakenings, decreased sleep time with associated daytime sleepiness, and impaired cognition in patients with asthma.[7,8] The resulting sleep deprivation may be associated with impaired ventilatory drive and contribute to the worsening of hypoxemia and hypercapnia in severe acute attacks.

Patients with CF may have more severe sleep disruption than in other obstructive lung diseases, resulting in impaired daytime functioning. Dancey and associates[9] reported that 19 patients with severe CF had reduced sleep efficiency (71%) and frequent awakenings, as well as lower mean saturated oxygen levels (Sao_2) when compared with ten healthy controls. Furthermore, the CF patients were sleepier, with reduced sleep latency on multiple sleep latency testing (MSLT) (6.7 minutes). These findings correlated with more reported fatigue and lower levels of happiness and daytime activity as well as impaired cognitive function.

Obstructive sleep apnea

The physiologic impact of OSA is well known. Patients become fatigued and sleepy, decreasing productivity and enjoyment of activities, while increasing the risk of accidents and injuries. Obstructive sleep apnea increases blood pressure and is associated with an increased risk of heart attack and stroke.

The relationship between OSA and insomnia is much less well described. The arousals and sleep fragmentation associated with apnea can result in sleep maintenance insomnia. More recently, the authors have identified a frequent compliant of sleep onset insomnia associated with OSA. This appears to relate to conditioning secondary to the significant sleep fragmentation associated with sleep apnea.

Clinical Management

Chronic obstructive pulmonary disease

Anticholinergics (ipratropium bromide), short- and long-acting beta agonists, and steroids are the foundation of therapy for COPD.[1,6,10] The recently available long-acting anticholinergic tiotropium may also be a useful nocturnal bronchodilator. These agents have a stimulatory effect and can therefore disrupt sleep. Because the disease process itself can also result in insomnia, careful attention to medication dosing schedules is necessary to minimize insomnia. Steroids should be administered in the morning, and the dosing of other agents at bedtime should be limited to those patients who have shown significant worsening of their symptoms at night. Albuterol and steroids can increase symptoms of restless legs syndrome, which, in turn, exacerbate complaints of insomnia.

Theophylline has been of interest because of its known beneficial effects on diaphragmatic contraction, central respiratory stimulation, and reduction of airway obstruction and gas trapping.[11] Berry and co-workers[11] compared a shorter-acting beta agonist with the combination of the beta agonist and sustained-action theophylline on sleep and breathing in patients with COPD. The addition of theophylline was found to improve morning FEV_1, non-REM oxygen saturation, and transcutaneous partial pressure CO_2, without impairing sleep quality. Unfortunately, sleep quality can be diminished in individual patients sensitive to the central stimulatory effects of theophylline.[11]

Asthma and other obstructive pulmonary diseases

In the asthmatic patient with persistent nocturnal symptoms despite adequate inhaled corticosteroid therapy, specialized intervention in the form of long-acting medications, such as theophylline and long-acting beta agonists, may be needed.[7,8] Inhaled agents such as formoterol, bitolterol, and salmeterol have been shown to improve nocturnal symptoms, increase overnight peak flow rates, and improve sleep in asthma patients. Although theophylline itself may have a deleterious effect on sleep quality, this side effect is somewhat balanced by the improvement in lung function in nocturnal asthma. One study comparing salmeterol with theophylline found only minor differences in sleep quality with a slightly higher arousal rate in those patients treated with theophylline.[7]

Obstructive sleep apnea

Continuous positive airway pressure (CPAP) management is the mainstay of treatment for OSA. CPAP improves nocturnal breathing and decreases the arousals and awakenings associated with apnea. The trade-off is that CPAP can result in sleep onset insomnia related to poor mask and pressure tolerance. Less frequently, mask intolerance can result in sleep fragmentation. Effective management of OSA requires aggressive and effective management of the insomnia related to sleep apnea and its treatments.

RESTRICTIVE LUNG DISEASES
Interstitial Lung Diseases

Restrictive lung diseases have traditionally been divided into intrinsic disorders involving the pulmonary parenchyma and those that involve the chest wall and neuromuscular systems. Dyspnea is the predominate symptom and it may begin abruptly or more insidiously with exertion. Dyspnea is progressive and may be present for greater than 6 months before presentation. Patients may present with paroxysms of dry cough that are refractory to antitussive medications, which can also worsen insomnia.

Sleep is disrupted in patients with interstitial lung disease. Decreased sleep efficiency and increased awakenings are common and may lead to complaints of fatigue or sleepiness, even in the absence of other sleep disorders such as OSA or restless legs.[12] This occurs along with a decrease in respiratory rate on falling asleep.[13] Furthermore, they have more time spent in stage 1 sleep, decreased REM, and increased arousals at a mean of 23.4 per hour when compared with age- and sex-matched control subjects who had a mean of 13.7 per hour.[14] Clark and colleagues[12] showed that in 48 patients, nocturnal hypoxemia was associated with decreased energy levels and impaired daytime social and physical functioning, and these effects were independent of

pulmonary function, as measured by the forced expiratory volume.

Neuromuscular and Chest Wall Disorders

The extrinsic neuromuscular diseases and disorders represent distinct challenges for the sleep physician. Sleep in neuromuscular and chest wall disorders were discussed in earlier chapters.

Behavioral Management of Insomnia

The impact of the co-occurrence of chronic illnesses such as respiratory diseases and insomnia is known to be detrimentally greater than the chronic illness alone on daytime functioning and quality of life.[15,16] In fact, chronic insomnia independently predicts diminished quality of life in persons with chronic mental and/or physiologic illnesses.[15] This fact is particularly relevant in the context of the large prevalence of insomnia, comorbid with chronic illness, which is estimated to be 60% of all insomnia cases.[17] Past assumptions regarded these cases of insomnia as secondary, or caused by the chronic illness, and therefore behavioral treatment was not expected to be effective for this population. Numerous studies have firmly established that cognitive behavioral therapy for insomnia (CBTi) is effective in alleviating primary insomnia, or insomnia in the absence of any relevant medical or psychiatric condition, however, the studies did not address secondary insomnia because many thought the best way to combat secondary insomnia was to target interventions toward the chronic illness instead of behavioral treatments aimed at the insomnia. However, as Spielman and colleagues[18] (1987) proposed, irrespective of the main, acute cause of the insomnia, maladaptive behavioral factors such as irregular napping and excess caffeine can maintain and worsen insomnia. In addition, actual diagnostic determination between primary and secondary insomnia is complicated by difficulty specifying cause and effect factors at work.[19,20] Therefore, it was argued that insomnia coexisting with a medical and/or psychiatric condition would be more appropriately labeled as comorbid insomnia, and because both medical and behavioral factors can contribute to the insomnia, behavioral treatment may be an appropriate intervention for this population.

A large influx of studies have now determined that CBTi is effective in improving sleep efficiency, sleep onset latency (SOL), and sleep quality across a variety of medical and psychiatric conditions without any additional intervention targeting the chronic illness.[21] Furthermore, the magnitude of sleep improvement due to CBTi is roughly equivalent regardless of underlying conditions.[21] Some of the conditions treated with behavioral interventions include: chronic pain syndromes, periodic limb movement disorder, post-traumatic stress disorder, osteoarthritis, cancer, Alzheimer's disease, alcoholism, and other serious mental illnesses.[22]

The first controlled clinical trial investigating the effectiveness of CBTi on a wide range of medical and psychiatric disorders also found significant improvements in sleep efficiency and quality; improvement was maintained at three-month follow-up.[19] Some other noteworthy examples include CBTi in chronic pain patients[23] and women with nonmetastatic breast cancer.[24] In both studies, sleep variables were found to improve both objectively, either measured by actigraphy or polysomnography, and subjectively. Lastly, Espie and colleagues[25] (2007) compared five sessions of group CBTi administered by primary care nurses to usual care in a primary care setting for a primary care population consisting of several conditions. Sleep efficiency, SOL, and wake time during the night were all found to improve and improvements were partially maintained at six month follow-up. Actigraphy also showed modest improvements as well as mental health, and vitality oe energy. This study suggests that CBTi should be a first-line treatment for insomnia in a primary care setting as opposed to pharmacologic treatment, and CBTi may also improve factors contributing to overall well-being beyond sleep factors.

Chronic obstructive pulmonary disease

Generalization of these outcomes to cases of insomnia comorbid with respiratory disorders is befitting, and thankfully several studies are confirming the effectiveness of CBTi for a few diseases underneath this umbrella of disorders. The first controlled study that included COPD patients compared the effectiveness of classroom CBTi, a home-based audio relaxation treatment with a delayed treatment control group.[26] CBTi was the most effective treatment in combating insomnia according to self-report measures, however, the other more cost-effective behavioral treatment also showed significant improvements on a few sleep measures compared with the control group. Unfortunately, actigraphic measures did not yield any significant improvements for either behavioral treatment, but self-report measures were maintained at four-month follow-up.

In an effort to make CBTi more cost-effective, Rybarczyk and colleagues[27] of the study mentioned above adapted the classroom CBTi into a home video classroom CBTi treatment with phone consultations. Twelve individuals were recruited including those with COPD and the results were comparable to the antecedent study. Not only did the treatment improve sleep efficiency, SOL, quality, time spent in bed, and wake time during the night, it also improved pain perception, mood, and social functioning. However, attrition was a greater problem with home-based CBTi compared with in-person CBTi.

The most recent randomized, placebo-controlled trial involving COPD patients was also conducted by Rybarczyk and colleagues.[28] CBTi was compared with a placebo group that received stress management and wellness training for patients with osteoarthritis, coronary artery disease, and COPD. CBTi vastly improved several self-reported sleep measures compared with the placebo group, and also improved daytime functioning according to a global measure. It was hypothesized that COPD patients would receive the least benefit from CBTi; however, COPD patients improved just as much as the patients with other conditions.

Obstructive sleep apnea or upper airway resistance syndrome

The first line of defense for these disorders has been sleep disordered breathing treatments such as CPAP, oral appliance, or bilateral turbinectomy. Insomnia complaints are highly prevalent in clinically suspected OSA at about 54.9% of all cases.[29] In many cases insomnia symptoms are greatly relieved by the treatments listed above. However, one study found that roughly half of insomnia cases comorbid with these disorders when treated with CBTi reached nonclinical levels of insomnia according to subjective insomnia, sleep quality, and sleep impairment measures.[30] When sleep-disordered breathing treatments were introduced after the administration of CBTi, most of the remaining patients followed suit. These findings further enhance the evidence that behavioral factors are involved with comorbid insomnia, and that they can be treated effectively with behavioral interventions.

Pharmacologic Management of Insomnia

The use of pharmacologic therapy for insomnia can be extremely challenging even in the otherwise healthy population. Patients with chronic respiratory diseases pose an even greater challenge. In addition to benzodiazepines, a number of medications from various classes have a potential place in the treatment of insomnia. Benzodiazepine and the newer non-benzodiazepine benzodiazepine receptor agonist hypnotics are prescribed frequently and, not infrequently, inappropriately. For example, one might mistakenly prescribe a hypnotic for an undiagnosed and untreated OSA patient who presents with an insomnia complaint, rather than ordering a polysomnogram. In the case of the patient with COPD, the patient may be better served by adjusting the pulmonary medications than by the addition of a sedative hypnotic agent.

The benzodiazepines and the non-benzodiazepine benzodiazepine receptor agonists both act at the benzodiazepine receptor (BZ-R) on the gamma-aminobutyric acid type-A (GABA$_A$) receptor, potentiating the effect of GABA binding to the receptor complex.[31] When GABA binds the receptor complex, it causes an opening of the chloride ionophore moiety of the complex. The resulting influx of negative chloride ions hyperpolarizes the neuron, thus inhibiting its ability to create an action potential. GABA$_A$ receptor complexes have five subunits (most have two alpha, two beta, and one gamma subunits) with the BZ-R located near an alpha subunit. The newer BZ-R agonists (zolpidem and zaleplon) preferentially bind where the BZ-R is associated with the alpha$_1$ subunit — so-called BZ-R1 agonists. The effect of BZ-R binding depends on the associated type of alpha subunit. When BZ-R agonists bind a BZ receptor associated with an alpha$_1$ subunit, they have hypnotic, amnestic, and some anticonvulsant effects but not muscle relaxant or anxiolytic effects. Thus, the selective BZ-R1 agonists have less muscle relaxant and anxiolytic effects than nonselective benzodiazepines. Therefore, when anxiety is a prominent comorbid condition, benzodiazepines may be more effective than the selective BZ-R1 agonists. Overall, both benzodiazepines and non-benzodiazepine benzodiazepine receptor agonists have been found to be effective in the short-term treatment of chronic insomnia.[32] However, neither of these pharmacotherapies come risk-free and the long-term efficacy and safety of many are still ambiguous.

The traditional benzodiazepines differ mainly in their duration of action (**Table 1**) but may have a variable effect on periodic limb movements. In general, longer-acting medications are more likely to have effects lasting into the waking hours, ie, a "hangover." On the other hand, some of the shorter-acting medications may be associated with rebound insomnia. Of note, despite some potential advantages of the selective BZ-R drugs, individual patients may respond to traditional BZs when they no longer respond to the selective BZ-Rs.

Although both zolpidem and zaleplon have a short half-life, neither medication causes prominent rebound insomnia[33] at least early in the course of use. Zaleplon has an especially short half-life and potentially could be useful as a middle of the night medication when a patient awakens but cannot return to sleep. A study by Walsh and colleagues[34] found a lack of sedation following middle-of-the-night zaleplon administration (testing 5 hours after drug administration) in sleep maintenance insomnia. One dosage of zolpidem at either 5 mg or 10 mg for COPD patients has been deemed safe in regards to respiration.[35] It also increased total sleep time and sleep efficiency with no significant differences between the dosages.

Although there is often concern regarding the possibility of physical addiction to BZ-R agonists, this is atypical in insomniacs unless there is a prior history of drug dependence. Physical tolerance to the drug and eventual ineffectiveness does occur in an unknown proportion of patients. Hypnotic-dependent insomnia is a significant problem, which includes drug dependency and a history of withdrawal symptoms. In general, all hypnotics should be tapered slowly to reduce rebound effects. A behavioral sleep program may also be helpful with hypnotic withdrawal. Other concerns include falls or other accidents from sedation or confusion from hypnotic use, especially in the elderly. It is always prudent to start with the lowest possible effective dose, especially in older or chronically ill patients. However, even at the lowest dose of hypnotics, confusion and sedation may occur in elderly patients.

The issue of tolerance is controversial because there are very few long-term studies of BZ-Rs. Certainly, some patients complain the medications no longer work well, but they may report a worsening of insomnia when the drugs are stopped. A study by Scharf and colleagues[33] demonstrated effectiveness of zolpidem over a 5-week period (no tolerance). Sustained efficacy over 6 months was also reported for the non-BZ drug eszopiclone in a large double-blind placebo controlled study.[36] In any case, some have challenged the conventional wisdom that long-term treatment with BZ-Rs frequently results in tolerance.[37] However, until more information proves otherwise, the recommendation to use hypnotics for as short a time as possible still seems prudent.

The other group of medications that are frequently used for treatment of insomnia are the sedating antidepressants. Surveys have shown that there has been a dramatic shift from BZ-R hypnotics to the use of antidepressants to treat insomnia.[38] Of note, unlike the BZ-R agonist hypnotics, none of the sedating antidepressants are FDA-approved for treatment of insomnia (ie, treatment of insomnia is "off-label"). In addition, the efficacy and safety of the sedating antidepressants as

Table 1
Medications used in the treatment of insomnia

Class	Medication	Half-Life	Onset	Dosing (mg)
Benzodiazepine	Alprazolam	Medium	Medium	0.25–2.0
	Chlordiazepoxide	Long	Medium	10–25
	Clonazepam	Long	Medium	0.25–2.0
	Clorazepate	Long	Rapid	7.5–15
	Diazepam	Long	Rapid	2–10
	Estazolam	Medium	Rapid	1–2
	Flurazepam	Long	Medium	15–30
	Midazolam	Short	Medium	7.5–15
	Lorazepam	Medium	Medium	0.5–2
	Oxazepam	Medium	Slow	15–30
	Temazepam	Medium	Medium	15–30
	Triazolam	Short	Rapid	0.125–0.25
NBBRA[a]	Zaleplon	Short	Rapid	10–20
	Zolpidem	Short	Rapid	5–10
	Esca	Long	Medium	1–3
TCA[b]	Amitriptyline	Long	Medium	10–100
	Doxepin	Short	Rapid	10–100
	Imipramine	Medium	Rapid	10–100
	Nortriptyline	Long	Medium	10–100
Triazolopyridine	Trazodone	Medium	Rapid	25–100
Other anti-depressant	Mirtazepine	Medium	Medium	7.5–45
Antiepileptic	Gabapentin	Short-medium	Medium	100–600
	Tiagabine	Medium	Medium	4–32
Dopamine antagonist	Quetiapine	Long	Medium	25–100
Other	Melatonin			0.3–3
	Ramelteon			8
	Diphenhydramine			12.5–50

[a] NBBRA, non-benzodiazepine benzodiazepine receptor agonist.
[b] TCA, tricyclic antidepressant.

hypnotics has not been well studied; however, there is some evidence indicating this group of medications is effective but not without risk of harm.[32] Some of the tricyclic antidepressants (amitriptyline, doxepin) that are commonly used as hypnotics have anticholinergic and cardiotoxic side effects. The antidepressant trazodone is not a tricyclic and is frequently used in low doses (50 to 100 mg) as a hypnotic. Trazodone is a serotonin type-2 receptor antagonist and a weak serotonin reuptake inhibitor. Although the drug does not have anticholinergic side effects, it can cause priapism, postural hypotension (alpha blockade), and morning sedation. Despite the frequent use of this medication as a hypnotic, the evidence of efficacy is scant. Yamadera and colleagues[39] studied the effects of trazodone on normal subjects with polysomnogram (PSG) and found an increase in stage 3 and 4 sleep but no decrease in sleep latency or increase in total sleep time (TST). Walsh and co-workers[40] studied patients with primary insomnia and found a decrease in sleep latency and an increase in TST with 50 mg of trazodone compared with placebo at week 1, but not week 2 of treatment. Sleep was quantified by self-report not PSG. The incidence of adverse side effects of trazodone at antidepressant doses is known but has never been studied at lower hypnotic doses. Nefazodone is less sedating than trazodone but is less commonly used after reports of the rare but severe side effect of hepatic failure from the medication. Mirtazapine is another antidepressant that can be used in low doses as a hypnotic. The most worrisome side effect of this medication is weight gain. Mirtazepine has shown some efficacy in the treatment of anxiety and post-traumatic stress disorder and poor sleep.

Other classes of drugs used as hypnotics include antiepileptics (gabapentin, tiagabine), antipsychotics (quetiapine), and selective MT_1/MT_2-receptor agonists (ramelteon). The antiepileptics and antipsychotics have not been systematically studied as hypnotics and can have significant side effects. The safety of ramelteon has been investigated with COPD[41] and obstructive sleep apnea patients in placebo-controlled studies.[42] At twice the lowest recommended dose, ramelteon was found to have no deleterious effects on apnea-hypopnea indexes for either population. On the other hand, the efficacy of ramelteon was poor for OSA patients, but COPD patients demonstrated meaningful increases in sleep efficiency and duration. As previously addressed, patients with depression frequently have insomnia complaints. Certain effective antidepressants (selective serotonin reuptake inhibitors [SSRIs], venlafaxine, bupropion) can also disturb sleep. If sleep complaints do not improve or worsen with treatment with these antidepressants, it is common practice to: (a) switch to a sedating antidepressant; (b) add a low dose of a sedating antidepressant at bedtime; or (c) add a BZ-R agonist at bedtime. Despite the widespread off-label use of sedating antidepressants as hypnotics, they would seem to be the agents of choice for the treatment of insomnia only where (a) BZ-Rs have failed, (b) drug-dependence is a major concern, (c) sleep apnea is present, or (d) depression is causing the insomnia.

In summary, chronic sedative/hypnotic prescribing can be a reasonable treatment option when a set of four preconditions have been met: (a) the insomnia is chronic; (b) behavioral treatments have been attempted and were either partially or completely unsuccessful; (c) sleep laboratory studies have ruled out the presence of untreated sleep apnea or periodic limb movements of sleep disorder (if there is clinical suspicion of these disorders) or if treatment fails; and (d) all sleep medications are prescribed by a single provider. When used, hypnotics should be prescribed in the lowest effective dose for as short an interval as possible.

REFERENCES

1. Petty TL. Definition, epidemiology, course, and prognosis of COPD. Clin Cornerstone 2003;5:1–10.
2. McNicholas WT. Impact of sleep in COPD. Chest 2000;117:48S–53S.
3. NIH. Guidelines for the diagnosis and management of asthma. NIH Publ No. 97-4051A;1997:1–80.
4. Turner-Warwick M. Epidemiology of nocturnal asthma. Amer J Med 1988;85(Suppl 18):6–8.
5. Turner-Warwick M. On observing patterns of airflow obstruction in chronic asthma. Br J Dis Chest 1977;71:73–86.
6. Ramsey BW. Management of pulmonary disease in patients with cystic fibrosis. N Engl J Med 1996;355:179–88.
7. Selby C, Engleman HM, Fitzpatrick MF, et al. Inhaled salmeterol or oral theophylline in nocturnal asthma? Am J Respir Crit Care Med 1997;155:104–8.
8. Swillich CW, Neagley SR, Cicutto L, et al. Nocturnal asthma therapy: inhaled bitolterol versus sustained-released theophylline. Am Rev Respir Dis 1989;139:470–4.
9. Dancey DR, Tullis ED, Heslegrave R, et al. Sleep quality and daytime function in adults with cystic fibrosis and severe lung disease. Eur Respir J 2002;19:504–10.
10. Douglas NJ, Flenley DC. Breathing during sleep in patients with obstructive lung disease. Am Rev Respir Dis 1990;141:1055–70.
11. Berry RB, Desa MM, Branum JP, et al. Effect of theophylline on sleep and sleep-disordered breathing in patients with chronic obstructive pulmonary disease. Am Rev Respir Dis 1991;143:245–50.
12. Clark M, Cooper B, Singh S, et al. A survey of nocturnal hypoxaemia and health related quality of life in patients with cryptogenic fibrosing alveolitis. Thorax 2001;56:482–6.
13. American Thoracic Society. Idiopathic pulmonary fibrosis: diagnosis and treatment. Am J Respir Crit Care Med 2000;161:646–64.
14. Perez-Padilla R, West P, Lertzman M, et al. Breathing during sleep in patients with interstitial lung disease. Am Rev Respir Dis 1985;132:224–9.
15. Katz DA, McHorney CA. Clinical correlates of insomnia in patients with chronic illness. Arch Intern Med 1998;158:1101–7.
16. Gooneratne NS, Gehrman PR, Nkwuo JE, et al. Consequence of comorbid insomnia symptoms and sleep-related breathing disorder in elderly subjects. Arch Intern Med 2006;166:1732–8.
17. Lichstein KL. Secondary insomnia. In: Lichstein KL, Morin CM, editors. Treatment of late-life insomnia. Thousand Oaks (CA): Sage Publications Inc.,; 2000. p. 297–319.
18. Spielman AJ, Saskin P, Thorpy MJ. Treatment of chronic insomnia by restriction of time in bed. Sleep 1987;10:45–56.
19. Lichstein KL, Wilson NM, Johnson CT. Psychological treatment of secondary insomnia. Psychol Aging 2000;15:232–40.

20. Ohayon MM. Prevalence of *DSM–IV* diagnostic criteria of insomnia: distinguishing insomnia related to mental disorders from sleep disorders. J Psychiatr Res 1997;31:333–46.

21. Lichstein KL. Behavioral intervention for special insomnia populations: hypnotic-dependent insomnia and comorbid insomnia. Sleep Med 2006;7S1:S27–31.

22. Stepanski EJ, Rybarczyk B. Emerging research on the treatment and etiology of secondary or comorbid insomnia. Sleep Med Rev 2006;10:7–18.

23. Currie SR, Wilson KG, Pontefract AJ, et al. Cognitive-behavioral treatment of insomnia secondary to chronic pain. J Consult Clin Psychol 2000;68:407–16.

24. Quesnel C, Savard J, Simard S, et al. Efficacy of cognitive-behavioral therapy for insomnia in women treated for nonmetastatic breast cancer. J Consult Clin Psychol 2003;71:189–200.

25. Espie CA, MacMahon KMA, Kelly H, et al. Randomized clinical effectiveness trial of nurse-administered small-group cognitive behavior therapy for persistent insomnia in general practice. Sleep 2007;30:574–84.

26. Rybarczyk B, Lopez M, Benson R, et al. Efficacy of two behavioral treatment programs for comorbid geriatric insomnia. Psychol Aging 2002;17:288–98.

27. Rybarczyk B, Lopez M, Schelble K, et al. Home-based video CBT for comorbid geriatric insomnia: a pilot study using secondary data analyses. Behav Sleep Med 2005;3(3):158–75.

28. Rybarczyk B, Stepanski E, Fogg L, et al. A placebo-controlled test of cognitive-behavioral treatment for comorbid insomnia in older adults. J Consult Clin Psychol 2005;73:1164–74.

29. Krell SB, Kapur VK. Insomnia complaints in patients evaluated for obstructive sleep apnea. Sleep Breath 2005;9:104–10.

30. Krakow B, Melendrez D, Lee SA, et al. Refractory insomnia and sleep-disordered breathing: a pilot study. Sleep Breath 2004;8:5–29.

31. Mohler H, Fritschy JM, Rudolph U. A new benzodiazepine pharmacology. J Pharmacol Exp Ther 2002;300:2–8.

32. Buscemi N, Vandermeer B, Friesen C, et al. The efficacy and safety of drug treatments for chronic insomnia in adults: A meta-analysis of RCTs. J Gen Intern Med 2007;22:1335–50.

33. Scharf MB, Roth T, Vogel GW, et al. A mulicenter, placebo-controlled study: evaluation zolpidem in the treatment of chronic insomnia. J Clin Psychiatry 1994;55:192–9.

34. Walsh JK, Pollak CP, Scharf MB, et al. Lack of residual sedation following middle-of-the-night zaleplon administration in sleep maintenance insomnia. Clin Neuropharmacol 2000;23:17–21.

35. Steens RD, Pouliot Z, Millar TW, et al. Effects of zolpidem and triazolam on sleep and respiration in mild to moderate chronic obstructive pulmonary disease. Sleep 1993;16:318–26.

36. Krystal AD, Walsh JK, Laska E, et al. Sustained efficacy of eszopiclone over 6 months of nightly treatment: results of a randomized, double-blind, placebo-controlled study in adults with chronic insomnia. Sleep 2003;26:793–9.

37. Mendelson WB, Roth T, Cassella J, et al. The treatment of chronic insomnia: drug indications, chronic use and abuse liability. Sleep Med Rev 2004;8:1–17.

38. Walsh JK, Schwitzer PK. Ten-year trends in the pharmacological treatment of insomnia. Sleep 1999;22:371–5.

39. Yamadera H, Nakamur S, Suzuki H, et al. Effects of trazodone hydrochloride and imipramine on polysomography in healthy subjects. Psychiatry Clin Neurosci 1998;52:439–43.

40. Kaynak H, Kaynak D, Gozukirmizi E, et al. The effects of trazodone on sleep in patients treated with stimulant antidepressants. Sleep Med 2004;5:15–20.

41. Kryger M, Wang-Weigand S, Zhang J, et al. Effect of Ramelteon, a selective MT_1/MT_2-receptor agonist, on respiration during sleep in mild to moderate COPD. Sleep Breath 2008;12(3):243–50.

42. Kryger M, Wang-Weigand S, Roth T, et al. Safety of ramelteon in individual with mild to moderate obstructive sleep apnea. Sleep Breath 2007;11:159–64.

Sleep Problems in Children with Respiratory Disorders

Mark Splaingard, MD[a,b,*]

KEYWORDS

- Respiratory disease • Children
- Sleep disorders • Pulmonary

Sleep is an active process associated with physiologic changes involving multiple organ systems. However, sleep can also be disrupted by organ-specific diseases altering the course of a particular medical condition, resulting in significant consequences resulting in a poor quality of life. Evaluation, assessment, and treatment of sleep problems in children with respiratory disorders is complicated by the changes in sleep physiology that occur in normal children from infancy to adolescents. These variations are important in deciphering the effects of respiratory diseases on a particular child's sleep. Generally the sleep problems in chronic respiratory diseases include upper airway obstruction, altered respiratory drive, or pulmonary mechanics that vary during the different stages of sleep, insomnia, or disrupted sleep continuity due to respiratory symptoms such as coughing or wheezing, medication effects, depression or anxiety related to chronic disease, or alterations of circadian rhythms. Several common pediatric respiratory disorders will be discussed in this article. Chronic lung disease of infancy (CLDI), formerly known as bronchopulmonary dysplasia (BPD), occurs as a result of acute neonatal lung injury and lung immaturity and may cause respiratory problems into adulthood. Asthma affects about 10% of children in industrialized countries. Cystic fibrosis (CF), the most common inherited pulmonary disorder, has a median predicted age of survival of 36.5 years with more than 70% of patients diagnosed by two years of age. Sleep problems in childhood lung diseases related to sickle cell disease (SCD), neuromuscular disorders, and scoliosis will also be discussed.

BRONCHIAL ASTHMA AND SLEEP

Asthma is a reversible obstructive lung disease manifesting as recurrent coughing, wheezing, and dyspnea in response to environmental triggers. Surveys indicate that prevalence rates in children range from 5% to 15%.[1,2] The prevalence is increasing worldwide with significant morbidity and considerable economic burden. Nocturnal asthma, characterized by diurnal change in forced expiratory volume in one second (FEV_1) greater than15% and asthma-related sleep disruptions have been reported in up to 80% of adult asthmatic patients.[3] Several adult studies have also identified that a significant proportion of asthmatic patients experience worsening of symptoms between midnight and 8AM, contributing to more emergency room visits, more calls to physicians, and greater proportion of asthma related deaths.[4,5] Although the prevalence of nocturnal asthma is not well studied in children, conclusions from the Childhood Asthma Management Program (CAMP) indicate that nocturnal awakenings occur frequently in children with mild-to-moderate asthma with 34% of children having at least one awakening and 14% having three or more awakenings each night.[6]

Significant worsening of lung function during the nighttime in patients with asthma is attributed to sleep or circadian events (**Box 1**).

[a] Ohio State University School of Medicine, Columbus, OH, USA
[b] Division of Pediatric Pulmonary/Sleep Disorder Center, Department of Pediatrics, Nationwide Children's Hospital, 700 Children's Drive, Columbus, OH 43205, USA
* Division of Pediatric Pulmonary/Sleep Disorder Center, Department of Pediatrics, Nationwide Children's Hospital, 700 Children's Drive, Columbus, Ohio 43205, USA.
E-mail address: mark.splaingard@nationwidechildrens.org

Sleep Med Clin 3 (2008) 589–600
doi:10.1016/j.jsmc.2008.08.003
1556-407X/08/$ – see front matter © 2008 Elsevier Inc. All rights reserved.

Box 1
Factors contributing to worsening of asthma during sleep

Increase in airway resistance due to activation of cholinergic pathways

Decrease in lung volumes

Enhanced airway inflammation

Nocturnal gastroesophageal reflux

Increased pulmonary capillary blood volume

Reduced mucociliary clearance

Diurnal variation in β2-adrenergic sensitivity

Melatonin secretion associated with increased production of proinflammatory cytokines

Normal healthy subjects experience circadian variation in peak expiratory flow rates that reaches a nadir around 4AM and a peak at 4PM. The amplitude of this temporal change is much greater in asthmatics.[7] Similar circadian changes have been identified in the cutaneous immediate hypersensitivity response to house dust allergen and in airway inflammation as documented by increase in inflammatory cells in the bronchoalveolar lavage fluid of patients with nocturnal asthma.[8,9] Sleep-related changes that can contribute to nocturnal worsening of symptoms include sleep-related decrease in lung volume, increase airway resistance due to cholinergic, and vagal mechanisms,[10] increase in intrapulmonary blood volume,[11] and reduced mucociliary clearance.[12] Temporal relationship between individual sleep stages and changes in pulmonary function are inconsistent.[13,14] The occurrence during the later part of the night appears to be more important than the particular sleep stage. Gastroesophageal reflux (GER) has been reported to occur in a high percentage of children with asthma and has been proposed to be a contributing factor for worsening of symptoms during the night.[15,16] The mechanisms that have been proposed for worsening asthma in relation to GER include vagally-mediated reflex bronchoconstriction induced by esophageal acid and microaspiration.[17] Reduction in leukocyte B2-adrenergic receptor density and function at 4AM compared with 4PM has been described, suggesting circadian variation.[18] The level of melatonin, a pineal hormone secreted at night that stimulates production of cytokines, has been found to inversely correlate with the overnight decrease in lung function in adults with nocturnal asthma.[19] Other contributing factors for nocturnal asthma include allergic rhinitis and rhinosinusitis. Not unexpectedly, the CAMP study also found

that worsening of asthma during the night is more prevalent in children with environmental allergies to indoor pets.

Poorer sleep quality has been reported in asthmatic children with frequent arousals, increased wake time, decreased mean sleep time, and reduction of stage 4 sleep correlated with asthma severity indices.[20] In addition, asthma symptoms and severity in children may be associated with impaired sleep quality and increased anxiety and depression in their mothers.[21] Poor sleeping patterns in children with nocturnal asthma can result in significant daytime consequences including poor school performance, attention problems, and neurocognitive dysfunction. Questionnaire-based studies attempting to establish a relationship between asthma and sleep disruption found that 47% of children with asthma reported night time awakenings and that daytime activities were affected adversely by sleep loss.[22] While the mechanisms remain unclear, neurocognitive dysfunction and impaired school performance has been recognized in some children with nocturnal asthma.[23,24]

Asthma increases the risk of snoring and obstructive sleep apnea syndrome (OSAS) in children.[25] Treatment of snoring and OSAS has been shown to improve the control of nocturnal asthma.[26] Sleep fragmentation due to nocturnal asthma may also affect respiratory control increasing the frequency of apnea in snorers.[27] Insomnia in a child with asthma may reflect occult OSAS and warrants investigation. Asthma is a risk factor for increased respiratory complications after adenotonsillectomy in children with a history of snoring and physical signs of upper airway obstruction pre-operatively (odds ratio -4.4).[28]

Since more than one nightly awakening from asthma symptoms per week is a criteria for at least moderate persistent asthma in children 0 to11 years of age, every effort should be made to optimize the control of nocturnal symptoms in asthmatic children.[29] Chronotherapy has been studied in adults with some evidence that an afternoon (3PM) dose of daily inhaled or oral corticosteroids is most useful in nocturnal asthma.[30,31] An evening dose (7PM) of a long-acting inhaled β2-agonist or once-daily sustained release theophylline may best control nocturnal symptoms.[32]

CYSTIC FIBROSIS AND SLEEP

Sleep complaints may occur in about 40% of children and adolescents with CF, with 70% reporting daytime sleepiness.[33] The degree of sleep disruption, measured by sleep efficiency on polysomnogram (PSG), was found to be inversely correlated with FEV$_1$ but not with nadir of oxygen saturation. While OAS may occur in younger children with CF,[34] it is rarely responsible for nocturnal oxygen desaturations in CF patients between 7 and 17 years of age with moderate-to-severe lung disease.[35,36] Pulmonary hypertension is well recognized in patients with CF without daytime hypoxemia raising the suspicion that nocturnal hypoxemia may play an important role. Neither respiratory muscle weakness nor malnutrition are necessary to develop hypoxemia or hypercapnia during sleep in CF.[37] The exact mechanism leading to desaturation is probably a combination of hypoventilation caused by changes in mechanics of breathing and derecruitment of ventilatory muscles, particularly in rapid eye movement (REM) sleep; and ventilation perfusion mismatching due to a reduction in functional residual capacity.[38] Oxygen desaturation is usually worse in REM sleep. Sleep hypoventilation with oxygen desaturation occurs with reduced FEV$_1$ (FEV$_1$< 65% predicted) or when resting oxygen saturation while sitting is less than 94%. Forty percent of these patients had oxygen saturation values less than 90% for greater than 5% of the night.[39,40] Although the threshold of nocturnal desaturation physiologically significant in CF patients remains unclear, adverse outcomes in right ventricular hemodynamics and survival in patients with chronic obstructive pulmonary disease have been reported at comparable levels.[39] Nocturnal pulse oximetry measurement should be considered in CF patients with moderate-to-severe lung disease even with normal resting awake oxygen saturations. Full polysomnographic study of patients with CF and mild lung disease may better determine what nonsleep study measurements will predict when patients first present with sleep disordered breathing.

Provision of supplemental oxygen at night to patients with CF, while improving some daytime symptoms, did not lead to improvement in survival.[41] Nocturnal oxygen therapy improved hemoglobin oxygen saturation levels during sleep but usually with accompanying increases in arterial Pco$_2$. Bilevel ventilatory support (BiPAP), with oxygen if necessary, was able to prevent hypoventilation during REM sleep and oxygen hemoglobin desaturation. Noninvasive positive pressure ventilation is effective in preventing sleep-induced hypoxemia in patients with CF and moderate-to-severe lung disease without modifying sleep quality and efficiency.[42–44] A recent report of a six week randomized placebo controlled trial of nocturnal BiPAP in stable CF adults with awake hypercapnia showed significantly improved nocturnal hypoventilation and peak exercise capacity, but no improvement in sleep architecture, lung

function or awake hypercapnia.[45] Further studies will be needed to determine whether survival can be improved with nocturnal support.

GER with abnormal pH probe is seen in up to 80% of children under five years of age with CF.[46] In contrast, a pediatric practice-based survey has estimated that vomiting, a common symptom of GER, occurs in 50% of non-CF infants in the first three months of life but in only 5% of normal infants at 10 to 12 months of age.[47,48] Hence infants and young children with CF are at a greatly increased risk of developing pathologic gastroesophageal reflux disease (GERD) that is associated with symptoms that include feeding difficulties, failure to thrive, recurrent respiratory symptoms including stridor, chronic cough and recurrent wheezing, and sleep disturbances. Proposed mechanisms for increased gastroesophageal reflux in CF are seen in **Box 2**.

Exposure of the esophageal mucosa to acid rapidly increases regional blood flow in tissue prostaglandin E2, and may cause inflammation and dysfunction of branches of the vagus nerve, which decreases lower esophageal sphincter barrier pressure, causing esophagitis and esophageal pain to worsen when lying in bed. Sleep as a state has significant influence on the physiology of upper gastrointestinal tract in normal infants and children. (**Box 3**).[49]

In contrast to the marked increase in swallowing following reflux during wakefulness, infants with pathologic reflux fail to increase their swallowing rate in response to reflux during sleep. Acid clearance time, which reflects the duration of reflux, increases from 1.5 minute while awake to 5.4 minutes during sleep. The secretion of saliva necessary for buffering refluxed acid is also

---

Box 2
Mechanisms of gastroesophageal reflux

Mechanical incompetence of the lower esophageal sphincter due to alteration of the shape of the chest wall and flattening of the diaphragm

Delayed gastric emptying and excessive gastric acid secretion due to abnormalities of pancreatic and duodenal function increasing enteroglucagon levels

Increased gastric pressure

Excessive gastric dilatation

Increased transdiaphragmatic and intra-abdominal pressure caused by forced expiration during coughing and wheezing

Transient lower esophageal sphincter relaxations allowing GER

Box 3
Sleep related causes of increased gastroesophageal reflux

Increased arousals or awakenings

Reduced swallow frequency

Decreased salivary secretion

Fall in upper esophageal sphincter (UES) tone

Supine positioning

Prolonged acid clearance time

significantly altered during sleep in normal children.[50] There is marked fall in UES pressure during sleep, predisposing to aspiration of the reflux contents.[51] A circadian rhythm of gastric acid secretion in normal children has also been demonstrated with peaks occurring between 9PM and midnight.[52]

A questionnaire-based study identified that non-CF infants and young children with pathologic GERD, compared with population norms, had a greater prevalence of nighttime awakenings, delayed onset of sleep during the night, and a greater prevalence of daytime sleep.[53] However, the propensity of infants and children under ten years of age to have higher arousal thresholds in slow wave sleep may make it less likely that children with GERD to have as significant sleep disturbances as adults.

There are data regarding the use of prokinetic agents and acid suppressive therapies in children with CF and nocturnal GERD, so a therapeutic trial may be justified in a child with CF and sleep maintenance insomnia with suspected GERD.[46,54–56] Nissen fundoplication for refractory GERD in childhood CF is controversial.[57]

Although prone positioning has been shown to be effective in reducing the severity of GER,[58] supine positioning confers the lowest risk for sudden infant death syndrome (SIDS) in all infants less than 12 months of age and is recommended by the American Academy of Pediatrics. While application of nasal continuous positive airway pressure in adults with OSAS resulted in marked improvement of nocturnal GER, no studies of this phenomenon exist for CF patients.[59]

Medications such as prednisone may cause insomnia in CF. It has been shown that children receiving ofloxacin frequently complain of insomnia, however, ciprofloxin is usually well tolerated.[60]

CHRONIC LUNG DISEASE OF INFANCY AND SLEEP

BPD was first described by Northway in 1967 as chronic lung changes that occurred in premature infants due to a lack of pulmonary surfactant.[61] This is now considered "old type" BPD because it generally occurred in 30- to 36-week gestational age newborns with respiratory distress syndrome (RDS) exposed to aggressive mechanical ventilation and high concentrations of inspired oxygen. The introduction of antenatal corticosteroids and surfactant replacement to prevent and treat RDS, along with changes in respiratory care strategies, have brought about a substantial reduction in this "old type" BDP. Yet, the overall prevalence of BPD has not changed due to the improved survival of infants born at 23- to 26-week gestation. The mechanisms of lung injury are different in this "new type" of BPD, since these infants may be born several weeks before alveolarization begins so that barotrauma and oxygen toxicity act on increasingly immature and more susceptible lungs affecting the normal process of pulmonary microvascular growth and alveolarization. The result is that the normal structural complexity of the lung can be lost with fewer and larger alveoli developing for gas exchange. Airways are more spared and inflammation usually less prominent than in the "old type" of BPD. Now BPD almost always occurs in infants delivered at a gestational age of less than 30 weeks and with a birth weight of less than 1500 g. Approximately 60,000 infants less than 1500 g (about 1.5% of all newborns) are born in the United States each year.[62] BPD develops in about 20% of these infants.[63] BPD is the most common cause of CLDI, a heterogeneous group of disorders producing acute lung injury that requires treatment with positive pressure mechanical ventilation and high concentrations of inspired oxygen during the initial weeks of life. Other causes of CLDI include pneumonia, sepsis, meconium aspiration, pulmonary hypoplasia, persistent pulmonary hypertension, apnea, tracheoesophageal fistula, congenital diaphragmatic hernia, congenital heart disease, and congenital neuromuscular disorders.[64]

BPD is defined as the need for supplemental oxygen for at least 28 days after birth, and is severity graded according to the respiratory support required near term. It is now the most common cause of CLDI in the United States.[65] Chest CT features like hyperlucencies, linear opacities, triangular subpleural opacities, and bullae are similar to findings seen in a presurfactant era (with the notable absence of bronchiectasis) and remain associated with duration of oxygen therapy and mechanical ventilation.[66] Currently, mild BPD is defined as a need for supplemental oxygen for greater than 28 days, but not at 36 weeks postmenstrual age (PMA) or discharge. Moderate BPD is defined as the need for supplemental oxygen for greater than 28 days posttreatment with less than 30% oxygen at 36 weeks PMA. Severe BPD is defined as oxygen requirements for greater than 28days plus greater than 30% oxygen requirement or positive pressure requirement at 36 weeks PMA. These consensus BPD definitions have been found to identify the spectrum of risk for adverse pulmonary and developmental outcomes in early infancy more accurately than other definitions.[67]

Studies now 20 years old showed that infants with BPD experience episodes of hypoxemia during sleep, even with acceptable awake oxygen saturations.[68] Episodes of oxygen desaturation values less than 90% were more common during REM sleep than during non-REM sleep. The degree of desaturation is correlated with airway resistance and linked to impaired pulmonary mechanics initiated by airway obstruction and inability to compensate for sleep related abnormalities. Episodes of airway obstruction and hypoxemia can further worsen the pulmonary mechanics of infants with BPD.[69] It has been shown that higher levels of oxygenation decrease airway resistance in infants with BPD.[70] Oxygen supplementation in infants with BPD can improve respiratory stability, decreasing central apneas and periodic breathing episodes during sleep.[71] Decreased oxygenation during sleep in infants with BPD has been associated with impaired growth. For instance, infants with BPD with oxygen saturations between 88% and 91% during sleep exhibited decreased growth compared with infants with oxygen saturations greater than 92% during sleep.[72] Severe desaturation episodes can be seen most commonly during REM sleep even in infants with awake oxygen saturations greater than 93%.[73] Infants with BPD have a reduced-total sleep time with sleep fragmentation and a decreased amount of REM sleep.[74] Sleep related hypoxemia may also lead to substantial impairments in right ventricular function and milder impairments in left ventricular function.[75] There is a well-recognized increase in mortality during the first year of life documented in children with BPD.[76] The higher incidence of SIDS associated with BPD may be in part related to intermittent acute hypoxemia and delayed maturation of respiratory control centers. There is some evidence that infants with BPD may not be at an increased risk for SIDS if they receive appropriate management including close attention to oxygenation.[77] Prevention of hypoxemic episodes in infants with BDP may well be the most effective means of preventing unexpected death in this group. Measurement of oxygen saturation during an extended period of sleep in these children by recording either plethysmograph waveforms or pulse amplitude modulation is important to distinguish true drops in oxygen saturation from artifacts due to movement or weak pulse signal.[78] While there is no clear consensus for the absolute threshold of oxygen saturation to be maintained during sleep, many clinicians target oxygen saturations greater than 92% during sleep to improve growth and respiratory stability.

A subset of children with CLDI, estimated roughly at about 5% overall, will require either tracheostomy or chronic mechanical ventilation at the time of initial hospital discharge. There is wide variation in this number between institutions due to variations in infants, family structure, and availability of local home care services. Polysomnographic studies done in children with tracheostomies can be very helpful in decisions regarding the degree of supplemental oxygen required during sleep. Determining the quality of sleep and the respiratory stability during sleep by PSG may be an important step before tracheostomy decannulation.[79] Home mechanical ventilation has been used in children with severe CLDI for the past 25 years (Fig. 1).[80,81] Polysomnographic studies may be very useful in deciding when changes in ventilatory support of children receiving home mechanical ventilation is indicated.[82] Since BPD is the most reversible cause of chronic home mechanical ventilation in the pediatric population, repeat sleep studies are recommended every 6 to 12 months to determine the need for and ability to withdraw ventilatory assistance. Recently, caregivers of ventilator-dependent children have been shown to have chronic partial sleep deprivation associated with depression and fatigue.[83]

Sleep-related GER may be a problem in infants and children with BPD for reasons similar to CF (see Box 3). However, current data does not show a clear causal relationship of GER and pulmonary disease in preterm infants.[84] No study in preterm infants has demonstrated prevention or improvement of CLDI with any treatment regime for GER and treatment trials showing improvement in outcome are lacking to support any causal relationship.[85] However, treatment for GERD is often instituted since it is possible that GER may be a contributing factor especially in some older children with BPD.

Sleeplessness may be a problem in infants and children with CLDI. A circadian melatonin rhythm is not present in term newborns and there is little evidence of rhythmic secretion of melatonin until 9 to12 weeks of age in full term infants.[86] Kenaway found that at 24 weeks of age term infants had 6-sulfatoxymelatonin secretion of approximately 25% of adult levels. Infants on average 51-days

A   2 years old   **B**   20 years old

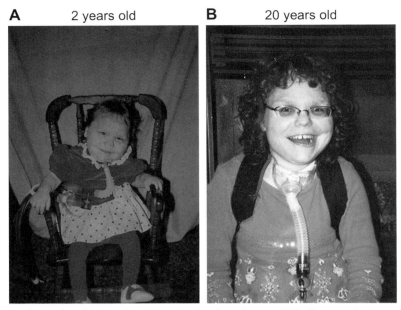

Fig. 1. Former 31-week 1.35 kg girl, born in 1987, who developed severe BPD. She was discharged home with tracheostomy, gastrostomy, and chronic mechanical ventilation at 23 months of age. At 21 years of age, she continues to require ventilator, supplemental oxygen, and gastrostomy feedings. *A.* Two years old. *B.* Twenty years old.

premature had a delay in the appearance of rhythmic 6-sulfatoxymelatonin of approximately nine weeks. Even after correction for gestational age or length of time at home, the premature infants were found to have a two to three week delay in the development of 6-sulfatoxymelatonin levels compared with full-term infants. A delayed peak of melatonin is associated with more fragmented sleep during the night.[87] There is also some evidence in normal adults that circadian rhythms apparent in normoxia are abolished by acute hypoxia.[88] While data about infants with BPD is generally lacking in this area, one recent study showed that infants greater than 27 weeks gestational age requiring mechanical ventilation in the neonatal intensive care unit exhibited immature sleep architecture with more active sleep compared with matched controls not requiring ventilatory support.[89]

Because the amino acid tryptophan is converted into serotonin and secreted in a circadian fashion, research has recently focused on chrononutrition in infants in an attempt to mimic circadian variations in the concentration of tryptophan to help consolidate the circadian sleep-wake cycle in infants. Cubero and colleagues[90,91] have shown that different day and night infant formulas designed according to the principles of chrononutrition may help to consolidate sleep-wake cycles in bottle-fed infants. Melatonin also has protective

action against tissue damage from free radicals and other toxins and may be important in prenatal or postnatal brain, ocular and intrauterine growth and development.[92]

SICKLE-CELL DISEASE AND SLEEP

SCD is the most common hemoglobinopathy, characterized by chronic hemolytic anemia and vaso-occlusive crisis related to the production of abnormal hemoglobin. Repeated vaso-occlusive crisis can lead to multiple organ dysfunction including acute chest syndrome, chronic lung disease and cerebrovascular disease.

Hypoxemia has been suggested as a risk factor for vaso-occlusive pain crises and clinical severity of SCD since polymerization of deoxygenated sickle hemoglobin is the primary molecular event in the pathogenesis of SCD. Episodic and continuous nocturnal hypoxemia is common and has been described in up to 40% of children with SCD.[93,94] Proposed mechanisms of nocturnal hypoxemia include OSAS secondary to adenotonsillar hypertrophy and SCD-related chronic lung disease. Extramedullary hematopoiesis and repeated infections are possible causes for tonsillar-adenoidal hypertrophy.

Although the exact prevalence of OSAS in children with SCD is unknown, Samuels and colleagues reported sleep-related upper airway obstruction in 36% and baseline hypoxemia in 16% of the patients with SCD (median age 7.5 years).[95] Adenotonsillectomy resulted in reduction or abolition of hypoxemia and decreased the frequency of vaso-occlusive crises.[96] Screening and appropriate management of nocturnal hypoxemia as a primary prevention of central-nervous-system events in SDS has also been recommended.[97] While a clear causal relationship between hypoxemia, OSAS and severity of vaso-occlusive episodes is not universally accepted,[98,99] it seems prudent to screen patients with SCD for OSAS and nocturnal oxygen desaturation hypoxemia using polysomnographic studies. Since the oxyhemoglobin dissociation curve for hemoglobin S is shifted to the right, a given oxygen saturation corresponds to a higher Pao_2 than would be predicted based on hemoglobin A. Children with SCD may have significantly elevated amounts of carboxyhemoglobinemia, so accurate determination of the fraction of hemoglobin bound to oxygen requires co-oximetry of an arterial blood sample obtained for precise determination of the arterial Po_2 rather than pulse oximetry. Adenotonsillectomy may improve symptoms of snoring and eliminate hypoxemic episodes in patients with OSAS. Children with SCD are at higher risk for postoperative complications after adenotonsillectomy. Preoperative transfusion before adenotonsillectomy to maintain minimum hematocrit of 35% has been recommended.[100] Currently, there is no data available to support the use of continuous nocturnal supplemental oxygen in SCD patients with nocturnal hypoxemia to reduce the frequency of vaso-occlusive episodes.

Pulmonary hypertension is a serious complication of SCD and was found in 46% of children and adolescents with SCD prospectively screened by echocardiography with a slightly higher odds ratio (2.8) in children with pulmonary diseases including acute chest syndrome, OSAS, and asthma.[101]

The relationship between daytime pain, nocturnal sleep quality, and mood has been incompletely characterized in children with SCD and further research is necessary.[102]

SCOLIOSIS AND SLEEP

Children with severe kyphoscoliosis may have significant sleep-related breathing problems.[103] In congenital scoliosis there appears to be failure of alveolar multiplication and in idiopathic scoliosis the alveoli do not enlarge normally. Cardiorespiratory failure attributable to scoliosis is usually a cause of death only in children who are first noted to have significant curvatures before 5 years

of age. It is rarely encountered in idiopathic scoliosis.

Respiration is more vulnerable during sleep for several reasons. All the respiratory muscles except the diaphragm and parasternal intercostal muscles are posture muscles. Therefore, breathing becomes entirely dependent on the diaphragm during REM sleep because the tone of all the postural muscles is reduced. Ventilatory responses to hypoxia and hypercapnia are most reduced in REM sleep. Spinal deformity itself reduces chest wall compliance increasing the elastic force that the diaphragm has to overcome to generate adequate tidal volume. Scoliosis changes the position of the spine and lower ribs so that that length and configuration of the diaphragm become abnormal and the force of contraction is diminished.[104] The diaphragm may also be intrinsically weak if the scoliosis is due to a neuromuscular disorder. These problems are compounded by reduced tone in the upper airway muscles during REM sleep. The upper airway narrows and becomes more collapsible when the diaphragm contraction generates a negative pressure within the airway during inspiration. Biochemical respiratory drive in scoliosis is usually maintained unless there is severe sleep deprivation due to repeated arousals from apneas or chronic hypercarbia, which blunts the ventilatory response. Patients with severe kyphosis cannot increase ventilatory activity because of a combination of mechanical and chest deformity, airway distortion, and depressed ventilatory drive.[105]

Nocturnal hypoventilation generally precedes respiratory failure diagnosed by conventional awake blood gas analysis and may be detected even when waking blood gases are normal.[106,107] Predicting which patient will proceed to respiratory or cardiac failure is imprecise, but for the clinician the best indicators are the level and severity of the scoliosis measured by the Cobb angle, forced vital capacity (FVC), the resting arterial Pco_2 during the day and night, and the presence or absence of muscular weakness.[108] While thoracic curves with Cobb angles as low as 80° have been associated with respiratory impairments, larger curves can be present without problems.[109,110] Hence, the degree of curvature alone is not necessarily predictive of sleep disturbance. Midgren found that nocturnal hypoxemia should be suspected if there is daytime hypercapnia or a fall in supine forced vital capacity of 25% to 50% compared with upright FVC, signaling diaphragmatic weakness. Patients with scoliosis frequently have severe nocturnal hypoxemia, obstructive apnea and hypoventilation.[111] Respiratory failure at night is most severe in patients with the most abnormal blood gases, probably because respiratory muscle weakness and decreased compliance of the chest wall and lungs are common to both sleep and wakefulness. The loss of biochemical drive and reduction in respiratory muscle tone make ventilatory failure more severe in sleep. Mean oxygen saturation during both sleep and wakefulness probably determines when polycythemia and pulmonary hypertension occur. The greatest oxygen desaturation occurs in most patients during REM sleep. Coexisting lung disease or obesity contributes to sleep problems. Sleep hypoventilation may be recognized by clinical features such as early morning headaches due to carbon dioxide retention, daytime sleepiness due to sleep deprivation caused by repeated apnea-induced arousals, or restlessness sleep due to movement or arousal. Personality changes correlate with the degree of sleep deprivation rather than the abnormalities in arterial blood gases. PSGs can be very useful in analyzing the severity of nocturnal oxygen desaturation, hypoventilation, and sleep derangements in children with kyphoscoliosis.

Short-term ventilation has been associated with a marked improvement clinical signs of respiratory failure in kyphoscoliosis. Children have been provided noninvasive ventilatory support at night using negative pressure ventilators, nasal BiPAP, or nasal intermittent positive-pressure ventilation. For many patients, ventilatory support is usually needed only at night to improve the quality of life and prognosis.[112,113]

NEUROMUSCULAR DISEASES AND SLEEP

Adults with spinal cord injuries often complain of sleeping problems and daytime sleepiness.[114] These problems are also seen in pediatric spinal cord injuries. Sleep apnea with excessive daytime sleepiness has been reported after spinal cord injury in up to 40% of adults and is more common in motor complete injuries and quadraplegics.[115,116] Children with spina bifida and Chiari Type 2 malformations are well known to have moderate-to-severe sleep disordered breathing including central, obstructive, and mixed apneas. Some of the patients require tracheostomy and mechanical ventilation due to central hypoventilation or upper-airway obstruction.[117] Sleep-related breathing disorders are common in Duchenne muscular dystrophy (DMD) with OSAS common in the first decade and hypoventilation developing in the second decade for reasons outlined previously.[118] There is a long history of treating children with neuromuscular disorders including spinal muscular atrophy, myopathies, and dystrophies

who develop chronic hypercapneic respiratory failure with a variety of different forms of noninvasive ventilation (NIV) or tracheostomy-positive pressure ventilation at home with improved survival and quality of life.[80,119] The evidence supporting treatment of nocturnal hypoventilation before the development of diurnal respiratory failure is limited. A multicenter randomized controlled study of preventive nocturnal positive pressure NIV in patients with DMD and moderate pulmonary insufficiency showed worse survival in ventilated patients in spite of improved daytime blood gases.[120] A subsequent randomized controlled trial of NIV for nocturnal hypoventilation in patients with daytime normocapnia showed progression of most patients to diurnal hypercapnia within two years.[121] A recent Cochrane review of nocturnal mechanical ventilation in patients with neuromuscular and chest wall disorders reports a weak but consistent therapeutic benefit.[122]

Children with myotonic dystrophy type 1 (MD1) have frequent complaints of fatigue and sleepiness and a recent study found almost 30% had sleep apnea and almost 40% had excessive periodic limb movements fragmenting sleep.[123] The decreased cerebrospinal fluid hypocretin levels and abnormal multiple sleep latency tests reported in some adults with MD1 have not been yet reported in children.[124]

REFERENCES

1. Crain EF, Weiss KB, Bijur PE, et al. An estimate of the prevalence of asthma and wheezing among inner-city children. Pediatrics 1994;94(3):356–62.
2. Smith JM. The prevalence of asthma and wheezing in children. Br J Dis Chest 1976;70(2):73–7.
3. Fitzpatrick MF, Engleman H, Whyte KF, et al. Morbidity in nocturnal asthma: sleep quality and daytime cognitive performance. Thorax 1991;46(8):569–73.
4. Horn CR, Clark TJ, Cochrane GM. Is there a circadian variation in respiratory morbidity? Br J Dis Chest 1987;81(3):248–51.
5. Douglas NJ. Asthma at night. Clin Chest Med 1985; 6(4):663–74.
6. Strunk RC, Sternberg AL, Bacharier LB, et al. Nocturnal awakening caused by asthma in children with mild-to-moderate asthma in the childhood asthma management program. J Allergy Clin Immunol 2002;110(3):395–403.
7. Hetzel MR. Circadian rhythms in respiration in health and disease with special reference to nocturnal asthma. Bull Eur Physiopathol Respir 1987; 23(5):536.
8. Mohiuddin AA, Martin RJ. Circadian basis of the late asthmatic response. Am Rev Respir Dis 1990; 142(5):1153–7.

9. Martin RJ, Cicutto LC, Smith HR, et al. Airways inflammation in nocturnal asthma. Am Rev Respir Dis 1991;143(2):351–7.

10. Haxhiu MA, Rust CF, Brooks C, et al. CNS determinants of sleep-related worsening of airway functions: implications for nocturnal asthma. Respir Physiol Neurobiol 2006;151(1):1–30.

11. Desjardin JA, Sutarik JM, Suh BY, et al. Influence of sleep on pulmonary capillary volume in normal and asthmatic subjects. Am J Respir Crit Care Med 1995;152(1):193–8.

12. Hasani A, Agnew JE, Pavia D, et al. Effect of oral bronchodilators on lung mucociliary clearance during sleep in patients with asthma. Thorax 1993;48(3):287–9.

13. Kales A, Kales JD, Sly RM, et al. Sleep patterns of asthmatic children: all-night electroencephalographic studies. J Allergy 1970;46(5):300–8.

14. Montplaisir J, Walsh J, Malo JL. Nocturnal asthma: features of attacks, sleep, and breathing patterns. Am Rev Respir Dis 1982;125(1):18–22.

15. Euler AR, Byrne WJ, Ament ME, et al. Recurrent pulmonary disease in children: a complication of gastroesophageal reflux. Pediatrics 1979;63(1):47–51.

16. Shapiro GG, Christie DL. Gastroesophageal reflux in steroid-dependent asthmatic youths. Pediatrics 1979;63(2):207–12.

17. Davis RS, Larsen GL, Grunstein MM. Respiratory response to intraesophageal acid infusion in asthmatic children during sleep. J Allergy Clin Immunol 1983;72(4):393–8.

18. Szefler SJ, Ando R, Cicutto LC, et al. Plasma histamine, epinephrine, cortisol, and leukocyte beta-adrenergic receptors in nocturnal asthma. Clin Pharmacol Ther 1991;49(1):59–68.

19. Sutherland ER, Ellison MC, Kraft M, et al. Elevated serum melatonin is associated with the nocturnal worsening of asthma. J Allergy Clin Immunol 2003;112(3):513–7.

20. Sadeh A, Horowitz I, Wolach-Benodis L, et al. Sleep and pulmonary function in children with well-controlled, stable asthma. Sleep 1998;21(4):379–84.

21. Yuksel H, Sogut A, Yilmaz O, et al. Evaluation of sleep quality and anxiety-depression parameters in asthmatic children and their mothers. Respir Med 2007;101(12):2550–4.

22. Meijer AM, Griffioen RW, van Nierop JC, et al. Intractable or uncontrolled asthma: psychosocial factors. J Asthma 1995;32(4):265–74.

23. Annett RD, Bender BG. Neuropsychological dysfunction in asthmatic children. Neuropsychol Rev 1994;4(2):91–115.

24. Dunleavy RA. Neuropsychological correlates of asthma: effect of hypoxia or drugs? J Consult Clin Psychol 1981;49(1):137.

25. Redline S, Tishler PV, Schluchter M, et al. Risk factors for sleep-disordered breathing in children. Associations with obesity, race, and respiratory problems. Am J Respir Crit Care Med 1999;159(5 Pt 1):1527–32.

26. Chan CS, Woolcock AJ, Sullivan CE. Nocturnal asthma: role of snoring and obstructive sleep apnea. Am Rev Respir Dis 1988;137(6):1502–4.

27. Levine B, Roehrs T, Stepanski E, et al. Fragmenting sleep diminishes its recuperative value. Sleep 1987;10(6):590–9.

28. Kalra M, Buncher R, Amin RS. Asthma as a risk factor for respiratory complications after adenotonsillectomy in children with obstructive breathing during sleep. Ann Allergy Asthma Immunol 2005; 94(5):549–52.

29. National Heart, Lung and Blood Institute. National Asthma Education and Prevention Program. Expert Panel Report 3: Guidelines for the Diagnosis and Management of Asthma 2007.

30. Beam WR, Weiner DE, Martin RJ. Timing of prednisone and alterations of airways inflammation in nocturnal asthma. Am Rev Respir Dis 1992; 146(6):1524–30.

31. Pincus DJ, Humeston TR, Martin RJ. Further studies on the chronotherapy of asthma with inhaled steroids: the effect of dosage timing on drug efficacy. J Allergy Clin Immunol 1997;100(6 Pt 1): 771–4.

32. Martin RJ, Cicutto LC, Ballard RD, et al. Circadian variations in theophylline concentrations and the treatment of nocturnal asthma. Am Rev Respir Dis 1989;139(2):475–8.

33. Naqvi SK, Sotelo C, Murry L, et al. Sleep architecture in children and adolescents with cystic fibrosis and the association with severity of lung disease. Sleep Breath 2008;12(1):77–83.

34. Hayes D Jr. Obstructive sleep apnea syndrome: a potential cause of lower airway obstruction in cystic fibrosis. Sleep Med 2006;7(1):73–5.

35. Jokic R, Fitzpatrick MF. Obstructive lung disease and sleep. Med Clin North Am 1996;80(4):821–50.

36. Avital A, Sanchez I, Holbrow J, et al. Effect of theophylline on lung function tests, sleep quality, and nighttime SaO2 in children with cystic fibrosis. Am Rev Respir Dis 1991;144(6):1245–9.

37. Bradley S, Solin P, Wilson J, et al. Hypoxemia and hypercapnia during exercise and sleep in patients with cystic fibrosis. Chest 1999;116(3):647–54.

38. Ballard RD, Sutarik JM, Clover CW, et al. Effects of non-REM sleep on ventilation and respiratory mechanics in adults with cystic fibrosis. Am J Respir Crit Care Med 1996;153(1):266–71.

39. Frangolias DD, Wilcox PG. Predictability of oxygen desaturation during sleep in patients with cystic fibrosis: clinical, spirometric, and exercise parameters. Chest 2001;119(2):434–41.

40. Versteegh FG, Bogaard JM, Raatgever JW, et al. Relationship between airway obstruction, desaturation during exercise and nocturnal hypoxaemia in cystic fibrosis patients. Eur Respir J 1990;3(1):68–73.

41. Zinman R, Corey M, Coates AL, et al. Nocturnal home oxygen in the treatment of hypoxemic cystic fibrosis patients. J Pediatr 1989;114(3):368–77.

42. Milross MA, Piper AJ, Norman M, et al. Low-flow oxygen and bilevel ventilatory support: effects on ventilation during sleep in cystic fibrosis. Am J Respir Crit Care Med 2001;163(1):129–34.

43. Regnis JA, Piper AJ, Henke KG, et al. Benefits of nocturnal nasal CPAP in patients with cystic fibrosis. Chest 1994;106(6):1717–24.

44. Gozal D. Nocturnal ventilatory support in patients with cystic fibrosis: comparison with supplemental oxygen. Eur Respir J 1997;10(9):1999–2003.

45. Young AC, Wilson JW, Kotsimbos TC, et al. Randomised placebo controlled trial of non-invasive ventilation for hypercapnia in cystic fibrosis. Thorax 2008;63(1):72–7.

46. Malfroot A, Dab I. New insights on gastro-oesophageal reflux in cystic fibrosis by longitudinal follow up. Arch Dis Child 1991;66(11):1339–45.

47. Nelson SP, Chen EH, Syniar GM, et al. One-year follow-up of symptoms of gastroesophageal reflux during infancy. Pediatric Practice Research Group. Pediatrics 1998;102(6):E67.

48. Nelson SP, Chen EH, Syniar GM, et al. Prevalence of symptoms of gastroesophageal reflux during childhood: a pediatric practice-based survey. Pediatric Practice Research Group. Arch Pediatr Adolesc Med 2000;154(2):150–4.

49. Bandla H, Splaingard M. Sleep problems in children with common medical disorders. Pediatr Clin North Am 2004;51(1):203–27.

50. Schneyer LH, Pigman W, Hanahan L, et al. Rate of flow of human parotid, sublingual, and submaxillary secretions during sleep. J Dent Res 1956;35:109–14.

51. Kahrilas PJ, Dodds WJ, Dent J, et al. Effect of sleep, spontaneous gastroesophageal reflux, and a meal on upper esophageal sphincter pressure in normal human volunteers. Gastroenterology 1987;92(2):466–71.

52. Moore JG, Englert E Jr. Circadian rhythm of gastric acid secretion in man. Nature 1970;226(252):1261–2.

53. Ghaem M, Armstrong KL, Trocki O, et al. The sleep patterns of infants and young children with gastro-oesophageal reflux. J Paediatr Child Health 1998;34(2):160–3.

54. Scott RB, O'Loughlin EV, Gall DG. Gastroesophageal reflux in patients with cystic fibrosis. J Pediatr 1985;106(2):223–7.

55. Rudolph CD, Mazur LJ, Liptak GS, et al. Guidelines for evaluation and treatment of gastroesophageal reflux in infants and children: recommendations of the North American Society for Pediatric Gastroenterology and Nutrition. J Pediatr Gastroenterol Nutr 2001;32(Suppl 2):S1–31.

56. Brodzicki J, Trawinska-Bartnicka M, Korzon M. Frequency, consequences and pharmacological treatment of gastroesophageal reflux in children with cystic fibrosis. Med Sci Monit 2002;8(7):CR529–37.

57. Boesch RP, Acton JD. Outcomes of fundoplication in children with cystic fibrosis. J Pediatr Surg 2007;42(8):1341–4.

58. Meyers WF, Herbst JJ. Effectiveness of positioning therapy for gastroesophageal reflux. Pediatrics 1982;69(6):768–72.

59. Kerr P, Shoenut JP, Millar T, et al. Nasal CPAP reduces gastroesophageal reflux in obstructive sleep apnea syndrome. Chest 1992;101(6):1539–44.

60. Upton C. Sleep disturbance in children treated with ofloxacin. BMJ 1994;309(6966):1411.

61. Northway WH Jr, Rosan RC, Porter DY. Pulmonary disease following respirator therapy of hyaline-membrane disease. Bronchopulmonary dysplasia. N Engl J Med 1967;276(7):357–68.

62. Birth: Final data for 2003. Hyattsville, MD: National Center for health Statistics, Centers for Disease Control and Prevention, 2005.

63. Lemons JA, Bauer CR, Oh W, et al. Very low birth weight outcomes of the National Institute of Child health and human development neonatal research network, January 1995 through December 1996. NICHD Neonatal Research Network. Pediatrics 2001;107(1):E1.

64. Jobe AH, Bancalari E. Bronchopulmonary dysplasia. Am J Respir Crit Care Med 2001;163(7):1723–9.

65. Baraldi E, Filippone M. Chronic lung disease after premature birth. N Engl J Med 2007;357(19):1946–55.

66. Mahut B, De Blic J, Emond S, et al. Chest computed tomography findings in bronchopulmonary dysplasia and correlation with lung function. Arch Dis Child Fetal Neonatal Ed 2007;92(6):F459–64.

67. Ehrenkranz RA, Walsh MC, Vohr BR, et al. Validation of the National Institutes of Health consensus definition of bronchopulmonary dysplasia. Pediatrics 2005;116(6):1353–60.

68. Garg M, Kurzner SI, Bautista DB, et al. Clinically unsuspected hypoxia during sleep and feeding in infants with bronchopulmonary dysplasia. Pediatrics 1988;81(5):635–42.

69. Teague WG, Pian MS, Heldt GP, et al. An acute reduction in the fraction of inspired oxygen increases airway constriction in infants with chronic lung disease. Am Rev Respir Dis 1988;137(4):861–5.

70. Tay-Uyboco JS, Kwiatkowski K, Cates DB, et al. Hypoxic airway constriction in infants of very low birth weight recovering from moderate to severe

bronchopulmonary dysplasia. J Pediatr 1989; 115(3):456–9.

71. Sekar KC, Duke JC. Sleep apnea and hypoxemia in recently weaned premature infants with and without bronchopulmonary dysplasia. Pediatr Pulmonol 1991;10(2):112–6.

72. Moyer-Mileur LJ, Nielson DW, Pfeffer KD, et al. Eliminating sleep-associated hypoxemia improves growth in infants with bronchopulmonary dysplasia. Pediatrics 1996;98(4 Pt 1):779–83.

73. Loughlin GM, Allen RP, Pyzik P. Sleep related hypoxemia in children with bronchopulmonary dysplasia and adequate oxygen saturation awake. Sleep Research 1987;16:486.

74. Harris MA, Sullivan CE. Sleep pattern and supplementary oxygen requirements in infants with chronic neonatal lung disease. Lancet 1995; 345(8953):831–2.

75. Praud JP, Cavailloles F, Boulhadour K, et al. Radio-nuclide evaluation of cardiac function during sleep in children with bronchopulmonary dysplasia. Chest 1991;100(3):721–5.

76. Iles R, Edmunds AT. Prediction of early outcome in resolving chronic lung disease of prematurity after discharge from hospital. Arch Dis Child 1996; 74(4):304–8.

77. Gray PH, Rogers Y. Are infants with bronchopulmonary dysplasia at risk for sudden infant death syndrome? Pediatrics 1994;93(5):774–7.

78. Lafontaine VM, Ducharme FM, Brouillette RT. Pulse oximetry: accuracy of methods of interpreting graphic summaries. Pediatr Pulmonol 1996;21(2): 121–31.

79. Tunkel DE, McColley SA, Baroody FM, et al. Polysomnography in the evaluation of readiness for decannulation in children. Arch Otolaryngol Head Neck Surg 1996;122(7):721–4.

80. Splaingard ML, Frates RC Jr, Harrison GM, et al. Home positive-pressure ventilation. Twenty years' experience. Chest 1983;84(4):376–82.

81. Schreiner MS, Donar ME, Kettrick RG. Pediatric home mechanical ventilation. Pediatr Clin North Am 1987;34(1):47–60.

82. Tan E, Nixon GM, Edwards EA. Sleep studies frequently lead to changes in respiratory support in children. J Paediatr Child Health 2007;43(7–8): 560–3.

83. Meltzer LJ, Mindell JA. Impact of a child's chronic illness on maternal sleep and daytime functioning. Arch Intern Med 2006;166(16):1749–55.

84. Akinola E, Rosenkrantz TS, Pappagallo M, et al. Gastroesophageal reflux in infants <32 weeks gestational age at birth: lack of relationship to chronic lung disease. Am J Perinatol 2004;21(2):57–62.

85. Jadcherla S, Rudolph CD. Gastroesophageal reflux in the preterm neonate. NeoReviews 2005;6(2): e87–97.

86. Kennaway DJ, Stamp GE, Goble FC. Development of melatonin production in infants and the impact of prematurity. J Clin Endocrinol Metab 1992;75(2): 367–9.

87. Sadeh A. Sleep and melatonin in infants: a preliminary study. Sleep 1997;20(3):185–91.

88. Stephenson R. Circadian rhythms and sleep-related breathing disorders. Sleep Med 2007;8(6): 681–7.

89. Hoppenbrouwers T, Hodgman JE, Rybine D, et al. Sleep architecture in term and preterm infants beyond the neonatal period: the influence of gestational age, steroids, and ventilatory support. Sleep 2005;28(11):1428–36.

90. Cubero J, Narciso D, Terron P, et al. Chrononutrition applied to formula milks to consolidate infants' sleep/wake cycle. Neuro Endocrinol Lett 2007; 28(4):360–6.

91. Cubero J, Narciso D, Aparicio S, et al. Improved circadian sleep-wake cycle in infants fed a day/night dissociated formula milk. Neuro Endocrinol Lett 2006;27(3):373–80.

92. Jan JE, Wasdell MB, Freeman RD, et al. Evidence supporting the use of melatonin in short gestation infants. J Pineal Res 2007;42(1):22–7.

93. Franco M. Sleep hypoxemia in children with sicle cell disease. Am J Respir Crit Care Med 1996; 153:A494.

94. Castele RJ, Strohl KP, Chester CS, et al. Oxygen saturation with sleep in patients with sickle cell disease. Arch Intern Med 1986;146(4):722–5.

95. Samuels MP, Stebbens VA, Davies SC, et al. Sleep related upper airway obstruction and hypoxaemia in sickle cell disease [comment]. Arch Dis Child 1992;67(7):925–9.

96. Sidman JD, Fry TL. Exacerbation of sickle cell disease by obstructive sleep apnea. Arch Otolaryngol Head Neck Surg 1988;114(8):916–7.

97. Kirkham FJ, Hewes DK, Prengler M, et al. Nocturnal hypoxaemia and central-nervous-system events in sickle-cell disease. Lancet 2001;357(9269): 1656–9.

98. Brooks LJ, Koziol SM, Chiarucci KM, et al. Does sleep-disordered breathing contribute to the clinical severity of sickle cell anemia? [comment]. J Pediatr Hematol Oncol 1996;18(2):135–9.

99. Needleman JP, Franco ME, Varlotta L, et al. Mechanisms of nocturnal oxyhemoglobin desaturation in children and adolescents with sickle cell disease. Pediatr Pulmonol 1999;28(6):418–22.

100. Maddern BR, Reed HT, Ohene-Frempong K, et al. Obstructive sleep apnea syndrome in sickle cell disease. Ann Otol Rhinol Laryngol 1989;98(3):174–8.

101. Onyekwere OC, Campbell A, Teshome M, et al. Pulmonary hypertension in children and adolescents with sickle cell disease. Pediatr Cardiol 2007 [Epub ahead of print].

102. Valrie CR, Gil KM, Redding-Lallinger R, et al. Brief report: daily mood as a mediator or moderator of the pain sleep relationship in children with sickle cell Disease. J Pediatr Psychol 2007 [Epub ahead of print].

103. George CF, Kryger MH. Sleep in restrictive lung disease. Sleep 1987;10(5):409–18.

104. Kryger MH. Sleep in restrictive lung disorders. Clin Chest Med 1985;6(4):675–7.

105. Todisco T, Grassi V, Ferrini L, et al. Respiratory function in scoliosis. Lancet 1985;1(8431):754.

106. Midgren B, Petersson K, Hansson L, et al. Nocturnal hypoxaemia in severe scoliosis. Br J Dis Chest 1988;82(3):226–36.

107. Midgren B. Oxygen desaturation during sleep as a function of the underlying respiratory disease. Am Rev Respir Dis 1990;141(1):43–6.

108. Branthwaite MA. Cardiorespiratory consequences of unfused idiopathic scoliosis. Br J Dis Chest 1986;80(4):360–9.

109. Sponseller PD. Sizing up scoliosis [comment]. JAMA 2003;289(5):608–9.

110. Weinstein SL, Dolan LA, Spratt KF, et al. Health and function of patients with untreated idiopathic scoliosis: a 50-year natural history study. [comment]. JAMA 2003;289(5):559–67.

111. Ellis ER, Grunstein RR, Chan S, et al. Noninvasive ventilatory support during sleep improves respiratory failure in kyphoscoliosis. Chest 1988;94(4):811–5.

112. Anonymous. Sleep and scoliosis. Lancet 1988;1(8581):336–7.

113. Bach JR, Robert D, Leger P, et al. Sleep fragmentation in kyphoscoliotic individuals with alveolar hypoventilation treated by NIPPV. Chest 1995;107(6):1552–8.

114. Widerstrom-Noga EG, Felipe-Cuervo E, Yezierski RP. Chronic pain after spinal injury: interference with sleep and daily activities. Arch Phys Med Rehabil 2001;82(11):1571–7.

115. Burns SP, Little JW, Hussey JD, et al. Sleep apnea syndrome in chronic spinal cord injury: associated factors and treatment. Arch Phys Med Rehabil 2000;81(10):1334–9.

116. Klefbeck B, Sternhag M, Weinberg J, et al. Obstructive sleep apneas in relation to severity of cervical spinal cord injury. Spinal Cord 1998;36(9):621–8.

117. Waters KA, Forbes P, Morielli A, et al. Sleep-disordered breathing in children with myelomeningocele. J Pediatr 1998;132(4):672–81.

118. Suresh S, Wales P, Dakin C, et al. Sleep-related breathing disorder in Duchenne muscular dystrophy: disease spectrum in the paediatric population. J Paediatr Child Health 2005;41(9-10):500–3.

119. Splaingard ML, Frates RC Jr, Jefferson LS, et al. Home negative pressure ventilation: report of 20 years of experience in patients with neuromuscular disease. Arch Phys Med Rehabil 1985;66(4):239–42.

120. Raphael JC, Chevret S, Chastang C, et al. Randomised trial of preventive nasal ventilation in Duchenne muscular dystrophy. French Multicentre Cooperative Group on Home Mechanical Ventilation Assistance in Duchenne de Boulogne Muscular Dystrophy. Lancet 1994;343(8913):1600–4.

121. Ward S, Chatwin M, Heather S, et al. Randomised controlled trial of non-invasive ventilation (NIV) for nocturnal hypoventilation in neuromuscular and chest wall disease patients with daytime normocapnia. Thorax 2005;60(12):1019–24.

122. Annane D, Orlikowski D, Chevret S, et al. Nocturnal mechanical ventilation for chronic hypoventilation in patients with neuromuscular and chest wall disorders. Cochrane Database Syst Rev 2007;(4):CD001941.

123. Quera Salva MA, Blumen M, Jacquette A, et al. Sleep disorders in childhood-onset myotonic dystrophy type 1. Neuromuscul Disord 2006;16(9–10):564–70.

124. Martinez-Rodriguez JE, Lin L, Iranzo A, et al. Decreased hypocretin-1 (Orexin-A) levels in the cerebrospinal fluid of patients with myotonic dystrophy and excessive daytime sleepiness. Sleep 2003;26(3):287–90.

Central Alveolar Hypoventilation Syndromes

Hiren Muzumdar, MD, MSc, Raanan Arens, MD*

KEYWORDS

- Central alveolar hypoventilation
- Congenital central hypoventilation syndrome

The ventilatory control system is tightly regulated. Three elements known to regulate this system include (1) sensors, such as peripheral and central chemoreceptors, and mechanoreceptors; (2) central controllers that receive input and integrate the response from the above sensors; and (3) effectors, including the muscles of respiration, that respond to the commands of the central controllers.

Thus, alveolar ventilation is regulated most of the time involuntarily by the respiratory centers located beneath the ventral surfaces of the pons and medulla, that receive afferent input from the sensors and control ventilation automatically (chemically) via the respiratory muscles. This chemical control regulates breathing during non-rapid eye movement (NREM) sleep. Voluntary control by cortical centers can also occur, particularly during wakefulness and during rapid eye movement (REM) sleep.

Central alveolar hypoventilation disorders denote conditions resulting from underlying neurologic disorders affecting the sensors, the central controller, or the integration of the signals. Such disorders can lead to insufficient ventilation and an increase in $PaCO_2$ (hypercarbia), as well as a decrease in PaO_2 (hypoxemia). The condition may be congenital or acquired, and affected children may be at risk from the neonatal period. Central alveolar hypoventilation may be present during sleep alone or in more severe cases during sleep and wakefulness.

It is important to make an early diagnosis of central hypoventilation to prevent the deleterious effects of hypercapnia, acidosis, and hypoxemia on cardiovascular and neurocognitive function. This review discusses the current knowledge on central alveolar hypoventilation syndromes, particularly in children, with special emphasis describing the recent knowledge about congenital central hypoventilation syndrome (CCHS) and rapid-onset obesity, hypothalamic dysfunction, hypoventilation, and autonomic dysregulation (ROHHAD).

CONGENITAL ALVEOLAR HYPOVENTILATION DISORDERS
Congenital Central Hypoventilation Syndrome

CCHS or congenital central alveolar hypoventilation syndrome has also been referred to as Ondine's curse and has been recognized in the literature for more than 30 years.[1] Ondine's curse (also known as Undine) was referenced to the story of a water sprite from European lore who cursed her unfaithful lover to lose all automatic functions and therefore stop breathing when he fell asleep. This rather apt description of the plight of subjects with CCHS has now become a part of medical mythology, but does not accurately reproduce the fable of Ondine.[2] The identification of associated features including Hirschsprung's disease, which is considered a neurocristopathy or developmental anomaly of the neural crest,[3] neural crest tumors, and autonomic nervous system (ANS) abnormalities has led to CCHS also being regarded as a neurocristopathy.[4–6]

Dr. Arens is supported by grant number HD-053693 from the National Institutes of Health.
Division of Respiratory and Sleep Medicine, The Children's Hospital at Montefiore, Albert Einstein College of Medicine, 3415 Bainbridge Avenue, Bronx, NY 10467 2490, USA
* Corresponding author.
E-mail address: rarens@montefiore.org (R. Arens).

Sleep Med Clin 3 (2008) 601–615
doi:10.1016/j.jsmc.2008.08.006

Subsequent work identifying abnormalities in a gene (PHOX2B) involved in the development of the ANS in the majority of cases of CCHS, if not all, has confirmed this concept.[7,8]

Epidemiology

CCHS is a rare disorder that is present across the world, with an estimated incidence of 1 per 200,000 live births in France.[9,10] Reliable estimates of prevalence in the United States and other countries are not currently available. The male to female ratio in many countries is reported to be 1:1.[9,10]

Ventilatory disturbances in congenital central hypoventilation syndrome

Ventilatory disturbances in CCHS have a characteristic pattern. The prominent respiratory disruption in children with CCHS is hypoventilation during sleep, although severely affected children may also have wake hypoventilation. Minute ventilation is reduced during sleep in CCHS because of a reduction in tidal volume with a relatively preserved breathing frequency. This pattern is much more apparent in NREM sleep when chemical control of breathing maintains respiration, than in REM sleep when a significant cortical component regulates breathing.[11-13] These findings suggest some type of alteration in chemosensitivity or alteration in regulation of the chemical ventilatory response in these subjects. Sleep hypoventilation results in significant endogenous hypercarbia and hypoxemia in CCHS, but these chemical changes characteristically do not lead to arousals and awakening from sleep.[4] Interestingly, arousals in response to exogenous hypercapnia are

relatively preserved, indicating at least some functioning chemoreceptor activity.[14] Paton and colleagues[15] found that the absence of chemical ventilatory control in CCHS extends to wakefulness with no change in ventilation in response to hypercarbia or hypoxemia in wake children (**Fig. 1** and **Fig. 2**). In addition, they reported a remarkable lack of dyspnea or discomfort in the children studied. The urge to breathe after a breath hold has been termed "air hunger" and the urge to breathe after exercise has been termed "shortness of breath." Shea and colleagues[16] found that children with CCHS did not have "air hunger" on inhalation of carbon dioxide and were able to hold their breath much longer than controls. However, if they were able to exercise heavily, they did reported symptoms akin to "shortness of breath." Ventilatory response to exercise in CCHS is abnormal: increase in minute ventilation commensurate with exercise is seen up to the lactate threshold, but beyond this level it tends to lag resulting in carbon dioxide retention and hypoxemia. This response is accompanied by lower increase in heart rate as compared with controls.[17-19] Shea and colleagues[20] investigated the importance of voluntary control of breathing in CCHS and reported that distracting mental activities did not compromise breathing in patients with CCHS, suggesting the presence of some mechanisms of involuntary ventilation. The ability of children with CCHS to increase minute ventilation in response to exercise is, at least in part, in response to movement of the extremities. Gozal and colleagues[21,22] showed elegantly that passive movement of the extremities, during wakefulness and sleep, induces increases in minute ventilation.

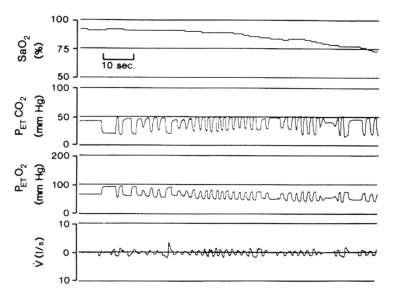

Fig. 1. Hypoxic ventilatory response during wakefulness in CCHS. Arterial oxygen saturation (SaO_2) inspired and end-tidal carbon dioxide tension $P_{ET}CO_2$, inspired and end-tidal oxygen tension $P_{ET}O_2$ $\dot{V}$(l/s), flow. Inspiratory and expiratory flow are plotted against time. There is irregular breathing without progressive increase in ventilation despite fall in SaO_2. (*Adapted from* Paton JY, Swaminathan S, Sargent CW, et al. Hypoxic and hypercapnic ventilatory responses in awake children with congenital central hypoventilation syndrome. Am Rev Respir Dis 1989;140(2):368–72; with permission. Copyright © 1989, American Thoracic Society.)

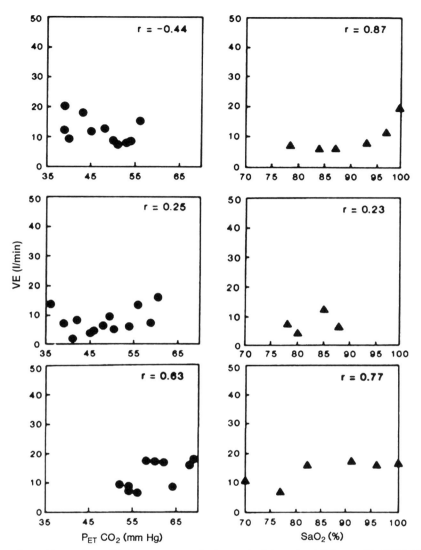

Fig. 2. Hypercapnic and hypoxic ventilatory response during wakefulness in children with CCHS. Minute ventilation (VE) is plotted on the ordinate. End-tidal (alveolar) carbon dioxide tension $P_{ET}CO_2$ is plotted on the abscissa for hypercapnic ventilatory responses. Arterial oxygen saturation (SaO_2) is plotted on the abscissa for hypoxic ventilatory responses. Each row represents one subject. There is no increase in ventilation with hypercapnia or hypoxia. (*Adapted from* Paton JY, Swaminathan S, Sargent CW, et al. Hypoxic and hypercapnic ventilatory responses in awake children with congenital central hypoventilation syndrome. Am Rev Respir Dis 1989;140(2):368–72; with permission. Copyright © 1989, American Thoracic Society.)

Taken together, these findings have led to the speculation that poor integration of signals in brainstem rather than affected chemoreceptor function explains the ventilatory disturbances in CCHS.[23] Using functional magnetic resonance imaging (MRI), Harper and colleagues and Macey and colleagues[24,25] studied the responses to hypercapnia and hypoxia and cold forehead stimulation (that bypasses central chemoreceptors) in subjects with CCHS. They reported significant roles of midbrain, cerebellar, thalamic, basal ganglia, and limbic sites in response to these chemical stimulations that are deficient in subjects with CCHS.

Autonomic disturbances in congenital central hypoventilation syndrome

Patients with CCHS have multiple disturbances of autonomic dysfunction including abnormal heart rate variability (HRV), attenuated increase in heart rate in response to exercise and increased frequency of sinus bradycardia and transient asystole.[18,26,27]

Reduced wake blood pressure and attenuation of the night time dip in blood pressure was demonstrated on 24 hour blood pressure monitoring in children with CCHS.[28] Pulse arterial tonometry (PAT) studies have shown reduction in the attenuation of PAT pressures with vital capacity sigh and exposure of the hand to ice cold water which lead to endogenous sympathetic stimulation.[29]

Pathology

Autopsy studies have not been contributory to the etiology of the disorder. Normal white matter or, in other cases, diffuse central nervous system astrocytosis, gliosis, and atrophy, but no primary brain stem abnormality, have been reported.[11] One report suggested small carotid bodies and an increase in lung receptors in two cases on autopsy.[30]

Clinical features of congenital central hypoventilation syndrome

Most cases present in infancy, usually in the newborn period, occasionally in childhood, and rarely in adulthood. Trochet and colleagues[31] have proposed that onset of hypoventilation after the newborn period (28 days of life) be classified as late-onset congenital hypoventilation syndrome. The common clinical features of CCHS are presented in **Table 1**.

Although most patients present with symptoms in infancy, some patients, including parents of children with CCHS, have been detected to have CCHS as adults.[31,32] Clinical clues to the diagnosis of late-onset CCHS include the ability to hold breath for prolonged periods without discomfort, episodes of cyanosis, daytime sleepiness and fatigue, unexplained seizures with normal electroencephalogram, evidence of right heart failure, apnea or delayed recovery after anesthesia or anticonvulsant therapy, and signs of autonomic dysfunction such as postural hypotension and low body temperature.[32] Late diagnosis is frequently associated with cognitive impairment.[32]

Genetics

Reports of CCHS in identical twins,[33] female siblings,[3] and male–female half siblings,[34] as well as mother–daughter transmission[35,36] strongly suggested a genetic basis for CCHS. A formal segregation analysis of ANS dysfunction in families of children with CCHS suggested an autosomal codominant inheritance pattern.[37] Initial studies focused on the genes that had known associations with Hirschsprung's disease, such as receptor tyrosine kinase, endothelin signaling pathway genes, and glial-derived neurotrophic factor.[8] These did not identify abnormalities that were seen exclusively in subjects with CCHS and were not present in control subjects.

The search was then directed to genes involved in the development of the ANS, and Amiel and colleagues[7] in 2003 reported heterozygous polyalanine repeat abnormalities in the PHOX2B gene mapped to chromosome 4p12 in CCHS subjects that were not found in control subjects. PHOX2b is a homeobox gene; it contains DNA sequences that are involved in the regulation of development. It has an early role in the promotion of pan-neuronal differentiation, repression of expression of inhibitors of neurogenesis, and regulation of the noradrenergic phenotype in vertebrate neural cells, including expression of tyrosine hydroxylase, dopamine β-hydroxylase, and receptor tyrosine kinase.[38–40] PHOX2b has two short and stable polyalanine repeats of nine and 20 residues (27 and 60 base pairs respectively) in exon 3.[7] Heterozygous expansion of the 20 residues to 25 to 33 residues (15 to 39 additional base pairs) is seen in most (about 90%) subjects with CCHS and is not seen in normal controls, suggesting a loss of function with the expansion.[7,41,42] Polyalanine expansions have been implicated in other inherited diseases such as X-linked mental retardation and seizures.[43] Polyalanine expansions are thought to function as spacers or protein-binding elements; expansions may thus lead to proteins that can bind DNA but have impaired functioning and interfere with functioning of the normal protein produced by the normal allele (a dominant negative effect). In this scenario, larger polyalanine expansions would result in greater phenotypic changes, which has been observed in patients with CCHS.[8] Reports of patients with deletions of the chromosome 4p region that included the PHOX2B gene but did not have CCHS provide evidence for a dominant negative effect rather than a haploinsufficiency model.[44]

The majority of PHOX2B mutations occur de novo, but Weese-Mayer and colleagues[8,42] have shown mosaicism for polyalanine expansion in 10% of unaffected parents of children with CCHS with transmission of the polyalanine expansions from affected mother to affected child. Other types of PHOX2b mutations that confer CCHS include missense, nonsense, and frame shift mutations in exons 2 and 3 and are less common (about 8%).[44] These mutations, in general, result in truncated or dysfunctional proteins with loss of protein function.[8]

Broad genotype–phenotype correlations can be made; mutations with a greater number of polyalanine repeats are more likely to have more severe disease (number of ANS symptoms), increased R–R interval, severity of ventilatory dependence,

Table 1
Clinical manifestations of CCHS

Respiratory	Nocturnal hypoventilation and daytime hypoventilation[4]
	Breath-holding spells
	Ability to breath-hold for a very long time with no discomfort
Cardiovascular	Cardiac arrhythmias including bradycardia, brady-arrhythmia asystole, decreased cyclical sinus arrhythmia[27]
	Need for pacemakers reported in 4% to 6% of patients[9,11]
	Reduced heart rate variability
	Vasovagal syncope
	Syncope
	Cold extremities
	Postural hypotension[98]
Gastrointestinal	Constipation without Hirschsprung's disease. Dysphagia
	Gastroesophageal reflux. Hirschsprung's Disease, about 15%
	Diarrhea without Hirschsprung's disease[98]
Ophthalmologic	Nonreactive/sluggish pupils
	Altered near response[49]
	Altered lacrimation[98]
	Strabismus[49,98]
	Anisocoria, miosis, ptosis[49,98]
Neurologic	Developmental delay[99]
	Motor and speech delay
	Learning disabilities reported in > 25%[9]
	Seizures (primarily during infancy)[9]
	Altered perception of pain[98]
Malignancies	Tumor of neural crest origin such as ganglioneuroma, neuroblastoma, ganglioneuroblastoma
Temperature instability	Altered temperature control
	Altered sweating
	Absence of fever with infections[9]
Psychological	Reduced anxiety[100]

and rarely, neural crest tumors.[8,42,44–46] Most of the limited number of cases of CCHS that have been shown to present later in childhood or were detected in adulthood have had five polyalanine repeats, the least necessary that has been shown to result in CCHS.[32,45,47,48] Nonpolyalanine expansion mutations causing CCHS lead to greater disruption of PHOX2b function and are associated with more severe ventilatory disruption, greater incidence of Hirschsprung's disease (87% versus 34%, respectively), and neural crest tumors (50% versus 1%, respectively).[44,47] Thus, Hirschsprung's disease and neural crest tumors are strongly predictive of nonexpansion mutations, and patients with nonexpansion mutations should be monitored closely for neural crest tumors. However, some frameshift mutations are associated with milder manifestations.[31,44]

The percentage of CCHS subjects with PHOX2b abnormalities had been reported initially to range from 40% to 97%.[7,41,42] This discrepancy may be related to incomplete analysis of the gene,

technical issues, or selection of patients that share the features of CCHS but may not have had all the ventilatory abnormalities.[44] In the largest series of 201 CCHS patients with genetic analysis, all patients had PHOX2b mutations, attributed to strict selection criteria for the diagnosis of CCHS.[44]

Diagnosis
Early detection of CCHS is important because of the significant morbidity, especially neurologic, and the risk of death in the undiagnosed subject. The American Thoracic Society published an official statement to increase awareness and promote early detection of CCHS.[4] The salient features of CCHS include (1) generally adequate ventilation while the patient is awake but alveolar hypoventilation with shallow breathing (diminished tidal volume) during sleep (more severely affected children hypoventilate both while awake and asleep); (2) better ventilation in REM sleep than in NREM sleep and progressive hypercapnia and hypoxemia with sleep; (3) absent or negligible ventilatory

sensitivity to hypercarbia and hypoxemia during sleep; (4) lack of an arousal response to the endogenous challenges of isolated hypercarbia and hypoxemia, and to the combined stimulus of hypercarbia and hypoxemia; (5) generally absent awake ventilatory responsiveness to hypercarbia and hypoxemia; and (6) generally absent perception of asphyxia (ie, behavioral awareness of hypercarbia and hypoxemia) even when awake minute ventilation is adequate.[4] Patients, particularly infants, may initially have only isolated symptoms such as extreme breath holding spells or temperature instability that may warrant further evaluation or careful follow-up. All cases of late-onset congenital hypoventilation should be tested for PHOX2B abnormalities. Of note, the diagnosis of CCHS is made in the absence of primary neuromuscular, lung, or cardiac disease or an identifiable brainstem lesion.[4]

CCHS can mimic many treatable diseases, and it is important to evaluate carefully for these conditions: (1) neuromuscular disease: discrete congenital myopathy, myasthenia gravis, or diaphragm dysfunction; (2) pulmonary disease: altered airway or intrathoracic anatomy; (3) cardiac disease: congenital cardiac disease; (4) brainstem lesions: structural posterior brain or brainstem abnormality or Möbius' syndrome; (5) specific metabolic diseases: Leigh disease, pyruvate dehydrogenase deficiency, and discrete carnitine deficiency; and (6) confounding variables including asphyxia, infection, trauma, tumor, and infarction should be distinguished from CCHS.[4]

The initial evaluation should include a detailed neurologic evaluation (that may require a muscle biopsy), chest x-ray, fluoroscopy of the diaphragm, electrocardiogram, Holter recording, echocardiogram, MRI of the brain/brainstem, and ophthalmologic evaluation to assess for pupillary reactivity and optic disk anatomy.[4] A rectal biopsy should be considered in the event of abdominal distention and delayed defecation to assess for Hirschsprung's disease.[4] Thorough airway evaluation (bronchoscopy, imaging) and evaluation of inborn errors of metabolism airway (such as serum and urinary carnitine levels or muscle biopsy for carnitine deficiency) may be necessary during initial evaluation.

The availability of genetic testing that identifies most, if not all, cases has made the diagnosis of CCHS much easier. A screening test for polyalanine expansion is relatively easily performed, and more detailed sequencing is indicated when clinical suspicion is high, and the screening test is negative.[42,47] Current information about genetic testing resources regarding CCHS is available at www.genetests.org, a National Institutes of Health–funded Web site sponsored by the University of Washington, Seattle, Washington. Most mutations arise de novo, but about 5% of parents have somatic mosaicism for a PHOX2B mutation and rarely have a germline CCHS mutation. Therefore, both parents should be screened for mutations and physiologically evaluated if they have mutations, and they should be regularly monitored even if asymptomatic. Children of patients with CCHS have a 50% chance of CCHS development, whereas children of subjects with somatic mosaicism have a less than 50% chance. Prenatal testing can be done if a mutation is identified.

Management

A careful evaluation of spontaneous breathing during sleep (NREM and REM) and wakefulness is essential to determine if the need for ventilatory support is during sleep only or during sleep and wakefulness. The change in tidal volume and respiratory frequency response to the endogenous challenges of hypercarbia and hypoxemia may negate the need for exogenous challenge testing. Before discharge, adequate parental training (eg, basic life support, tracheostomy care), backup ventilation, appropriate nursing assistance, and monitoring equipment need to be arranged. Pulse oximetry and end tidal carbon dioxide monitoring can provide objective evidence of early decompensation of ventilation such as with intercurrent infections, especially because this may be masked by the lack of dyspnea in patients with CCHS. In addition, these parameters can detect at an early stage the need to increase ventilatory support with growth.[4]

Ventilatory support

Ventilatory support can be provided by a mechanical ventilator via a tracheostomy, noninvasive ventilation via face/nasal mask, negative pressure ventilators, and diaphragmatic pacing. Ventilatory support may be needed continually or only when asleep.

Infants who require 24-hour ventilatory support will need mechanical ventilation via tracheostomy. With increased mobility, it may be feasible to transition them to daytime diaphragmatic pacing with a better quality of life. Speech can be attempted in children with diaphragmatic pacing with one-way speaking valves such as the Passy-Muir speaking valve (Passy-Muir, Irvine, California); readiness for speech may be assessed by capping the tracheostomy tube and allowing the child to breathe around the uncuffed tracheostomy tube. Periodic surveillance of the tracheostomy site for complications such as granulation tissue can help anticipate problems with ventilation, tracheostomy care, and speech with a speaking valve. As the child matures, it may be possible to manage ventilation with daytime pacing and nighttime noninvasive mask ventilation.

Children who require support only at night were initially been managed by tracheostomy and mechanical ventilation but now often are managed with noninvasive ventilation (NIV) with Bilevel Positive Airway Pressure (BLPAP) devices via a face mask. BLPAP ventilation is set up so that the difference between inspiratory and expiratory pressure generates adequate tidal volume with an expiratory pressure sufficient to maintain adequate functional residual capacity. A backup ventilatory rate is dialed in to guarantee minute ventilation. The use of NIV has become more widespread, and in an international survey of patients with CCHS, Vanderlaan and colleagues[9] reported that 14% of patients had never been tracheotomized and were managed by noninvasive ventilation. Children with CCHS who are maintained on nocturnal ventilation need close monitoring at the age of 2 to 3 years because they may have a greater need for wake ventilatory support during this time.[4] Adenotonsillar hypertrophy is also common at this age and may interfere with mask ventilation. Facial growth should be regularly assessed by craniofacial experts in infants and younger children receiving mask ventilation because of the potential for midfacial hypoplasia.

The suggested target for ventilatory support is to maintain oxyhemoglobin saturation at or above 95%. End tidal carbon dioxide levels in the 30- to 45–mm Hg range are recommended to provide a safety margin for adequate ventilation in the home environment.[4] A target level of 30 to 35 mm Hg at night has also been advised based on potential improvement in daytime ventilation brought about by mild nocturnal hyperventilation.[23]

Children who need only nocturnal NIV may be candidates for nocturnal diaphragmatic pacing that may become the sole mode of ventilatory support for these children.[23] These children may need additional daytime support via NIV or more aggressive support by endotracheal intubation in the presence of illness or lower respiratory tract infections. Diaphragmatic pacing stimulates the patient's phrenic nerves by an external transmitter, antenna, receiver, and electrode. The external transmitter sets the respiratory rate and length of inspiration. It transmits the signal and energy by inductive coupling across intact skin via the antenna to the subcutaneous receiver. The phrenic nerves are then stimulated by the implanted electrodes. The diaphragmatic musculature needs to be trained by gradually increasing the duration of

stimulation to overcome fatigue. Pacing is usually limited to 12 to 16 hours at a stretch, although 24-hour stimulation has been done.[23] Diaphragmatic contractions reduce upper airway pressure and have the potential to cause upper airway obstruction. Pacing equipment can malfunction, and a backup mode of ventilation is important as is proximity to a team that can manage the malfunctions.[23]

Negative pressure ventilators expand the chest and abdomen by external negative pressure. This can be delivered by an external shell (cuirass) or a wrap and is also available as a relatively portable product (Porta-Lung Inc., Lakewood, Colorado; http://portalung.com/). These ventilators are more cumbersome, limit access to the body, and may cause upper airway obstruction during sleep.[23] However, there may be an option for patients who do not tolerate positive pressure ventilation.

Long-term management

Patients with CCHS have so many special needs that it is advisable to coordinate their care with a center that has the expertise in managing CCHS.[4] These needs include the following:

1) Close monitoring of growth and development including detailed neurocognitive testing for impairments that may be caused by CCHS or is secondary to hypoxemia.
2) Regular echocardiography to gauge pulmonary arterial pressure and ambulatory electrocardiographic monitoring to assess for asystole, particularly with symptoms of dizziness and syncope. These evaluations may inform the need for better ventilation and cardiac pacing.[4,46]
3) Careful periodic ophthalmologic evaluation because of the high incidence of ocular abnormalities.[4,49]
4) A high index of suspicion for the management of infection in children with CCHS because of the impaired ability to sense hypoxemia, poor perception of respiratory distress in response to lower respiratory infections, and unpredictable temperature control. Management is optimized by objective evaluation of respiratory status by pulse oximetry and end tidal carbon dioxide monitoring and by well-informed, skilled, and consistent care at home.
5) Limitation of sporting activity to noncontact sports and to moderate exercise with many rest periods because of the potential inability to adapt to greater exercise loads and lack of recognition of hypoxemia, hypercarbia, and acidosis. Swimming carries significant risk and, if allowed, should only be done under

close supervision by a competent caretaker who limits submersion time and ensures frequent rests.[4]

6) Children with nonpolyalanine expansion mutations should be screened for Hirschsprung's disease and surveilled for neural crest tumors in infancy and childhood.

7) Close attention and objective monitoring after sedation and anesthesia is necessary because of the potential of prolonged apneas.[32]

8) Counseling and advising abstinence from alcohol is important because of the potential for adverse outcomes including coma and death, particularly during adolescence.[50]

Support groups can very useful to help parents and children cope with these unique problems.

Prognosis

The first few years of life are associated with the greatest need for medical attention, and long-term outcome is variable.[4,23] Children with CCHS do not outgrow the need of ventilatory support during sleep and remain technology dependant, and, internationally, support varies widely across various regions of the globe.[9] The long-term outcome of neurodevelopment with optimal ventilatory support has not been established. Overall, once the condition is identified, with appropriate support, the outcome has improved with a reasonable quality of life.

Myelomeningocele with Arnold Chiari Type II Malformation

Arnold-Chiari malformation (ACM) is a congenital brain malformation involving a deformity of the brainstem caused by herniation of the medulla and cerebellum through the foramen magnum. Arnold Chiari malformation type II is associated with myelomeningocele, hydrocephalus, and herniation of the cerebellar tonsils; caudal brainstem; and fourth ventricle through the foramen magnum. These patients are at risk for alterations in ventilatory control because of the involvement of respiratory centers located within the affected areas or involvement of brainstem nuclei controlling upper airway motor musculature and sensation. It has been speculated that both traction from the myelomeningocele and increased intracranial pressure caused by hydrocephalus may cause compression of respiratory centers controlling the ventilatory patterns. Alternatively, it has been proposed that a primary deficit in brain stem structure may be responsible for respiratory deficits observed in these subjects.

Ventilatory patterns during sleep

Sleep disordered breathing including obstructive sleep apnea and hypoventilation has been reported in subjects with ACM type II. The exact prevalence is unknown. A large report by Hayes and colleagues,[51] suggests that about 5.7% (35 of 616) children have evidence of significant central ventilatory dysfunction including vocal cord paralysis, stridor, apnea, hypoventilation, and bradyarrhythmia. In another study of asymptomatic patients with ACM type II, Ward and colleagues[52] noted hypoventilation in up to 70% of children. Interestingly, in about 30% of cases, these symptoms may be reversible once children undergo treatment for the hydrocephalus or decompression of the brainstem.[53]

Ventilatory responses

Significant blunted ventilatory responses to hypercapnia and, to a lesser degree, hypoxia have been noted by Swaminathan and colleagues[54] in children with ACM type II. These findings were also observed by Gozal and colleagues[55] who tested peripheral chemosensitivity in these subjects and noted a few with altered hypoxic responses. They have speculated that central ventilatory controllers may be affected in these subjects by traction of the ACM affecting integration of chemoreceptor output.[55]

Management

Presence of upper airway obstruction and vocal cord paralysis during wakefulness requires immediate medical attention. If not responsive to treatment of hydrocephalus or posterior fossa decompression, tracheostomy and mechanical ventilation are indicated. Children with significant hypoventilation during sleep or wakefulness will require chronic mechanical ventilation to sustain an adequate life quality.[53]

Prader-Willi Syndrome

Prader-Willi syndrome (PWS) is a genetic disorder resulting from a parental imprinting abnormality of chromosome 15 in the Prader-Willi critical region (PWCR). The prevalence of the disorder is estimated at 1 per 10,000 to 1 per 25,000 births. Clinically, PWS is characterized by mental retardation, severe hypotonia, and feeding difficulties in early infancy followed later by excessive eating and gradual development of morbid obesity. It is believed that a primary hypothalamic dysfunction has a major role in the disorder leading to hyperphagia, growth hormone deficiency and short stature, temperature instability, and hypogonadotropic hypogonadism.

Ventilatory patterns during sleep

Various studies suggest that PWS subjects are at increased risk for the development of obstructive sleep apnea, central sleep apnea, and alveolar hypoventilation during sleep.[56–58] However, the exact prevalence of sleep-disordered breathing in PWS is not well established.[58] PWS subjects are at risk for the development of such disorders because of obesity, alterations in cranial structure, hypotonia, restrictive lung disease, and altered ventilatory responses.[58]

Altered ventilatory responses

Ventilatory responses to hypoxia are absent or significantly reduced in subjects with PWS and are independent of degree of obesity.[59] In contrast, hypercapnic ventilatory responses were shown to be normal in nonobese PWS and blunted in obese PWS subjects compared with controls.[59] These findings are supported by studies showing absence of peripheral chemosensitivity in PWS[60] and studies showing poor arousal and cardiorespiratory responses to hypoxia and hypercapnia from slow wave sleep in these subjects.[57,61] Recent reports document sudden death during sleep in some subjects when treated with growth hormone to improve growth velocity and improve body composition.[62–68] Although mechanisms leading to sudden death have not been elucidated, abnormalities in ventilatory control and respiratory infections have been noted. Consequently, polysomnography before treatment with growth hormone and careful monitoring during respiratory infections is recommended.[66–68]

RAPID-ONSET OBESITY HYPOTHALAMIC DYSFUNCTION AND AUTONOMIC DYSREGULATION

The occurrence of late-onset central hypoventilation syndrome (LO-CHS) with features overlapping with CCHS in association with hypothalamic abnormalities was initially reported in 1965.[69] It was reviewed by Katz and colleagues[70] in 2000 when they noted this pattern of later age of onset and associated hypothalamic dysfunction (LO-CHS/HD), which distinguished it from CCHS. They also reported that early obesity/hyperphagia was present in all these patients.[70] Ize-Ludlow and colleagues[71] recently published a detailed study of 15 patients with LO-CHS, identified the consistent early presentation of rapid onset of obesity with associated autonomic abnormalities with hypoventilation, and coined the acronym ROHHAD (Rapid-onset obesity with hypothalamic dysfunction, hypoventilation, and autonomic dysregulation) to facilitate identification of this phenotype.

They did not find any mutations of PHOX2B or two other candidate genes, BDNF and TRKB, that are involved in neuronal development, in their series of cases. More extensive DNA analysis of two of 15 patients also did not reveal any abnormalities. MRI scans done in patients before cardiorespiratory arrest were not specific; one patient had Rathke's cleft cyst and another had hypointensities in the pons and medulla.[71]

Clinical Features

Nine girls and six boys are included in the above report with most having rapid onset of obesity as the initial manifestation followed by hypothalamic dysfunction, then autonomic abnormalities, and eventually hypoventilation. The median age for onset of obesity and hypothalamic dysfunction was 3 years, for autonomic dysfunction 3.6 years, and for hypoventilation 6.2 years. Hypernatremia was a common feature of hypothalamic dysfunction, and ophthalmologic abnormalities were seen in 13 of 15 children. A remarkable finding was the development of neural crest tumors in five of 15 children with this syndrome. A summary of clinical features is listed in **Table 2**.

All of 9 children tested had central alveolar hypoventilation with mild baseline tachypnea, hypoventilation, and hypoxemia during wakefulness with impaired response to endogenous hypercarbia and hypoxemia during NREM sleep. Seven of the 15 children reported required 24-hour ventilatory support, whereas the rest needed support at night. Of note, 60% of the children were reported to have cardiorespiratory arrest; some of these had some disturbances in respiratory function before arrest, including nocturnal desaturation, obstructive sleep apnea, and cyanotic episodes.

Diagnosis and Management

The diagnosis of ROHHAD rests on the identification of the rapid onset of obesity, hypothalamic dysfunction, and autonomic abnormalities and alveolar hypoventilation in children with normal initial first 2 to 4 years of life. Identification of the pattern of rapid obesity, hypothalamic abnormalities, and autonomic abnormalities is imperative to prevent morbidity and mortality associated with this syndrome.[71] Close monitoring of their ventilatory status is currently recommended at 3- to 6-month intervals in addition to periodic surveillance for neural crest tumors.[71] These recommendations for management may change as understanding of the molecular basis, pathophysiology, prognostic markers, and long-term outcome of this syndrome advances.

Table 2
Clinical manifestations of ROHHAD

Endocrine	Obesity of rapid onset, hyperphagia
	Hypernatremia, polyuria, polydypsia, hyponatremia
	Hyperprolactinemia
	Precocious puberty, delayed puberty
	Hypogonadism, amenorrhea
	Failed growth hormone stimulation test, short stature
	Hypothyroidism
Autonomic	Temperature control abnormalities, altered sweating
	Altered perception of pain
	Cold extremities
	Bradycardia
Ophthalmologic	Pupillary abnormalities and strabismus
Respiratory	Central hypoventilation
	Cyanotic spells
	Cardiorespiratory arrest
	Obstructive sleep apnea
Neuropsychiatric	Behavior disorders
	Autism spectrum disorder
	Developmental delay and regression
	Seizures
	Bipolar disorder, depression
	Psychosis
Gastrointestinal	Constipation
	Diarrhea
Neural crest tumors	Ganglioneuroma
	Ganglioneuroblastoma

OBESITY HYPOVENTILATION SYNDROME

Obesity hypoventilation syndrome (OHS) is an incompletely understood syndrome of central hypoventilation during wakefulness that is seen in obese patients with sleep disordered breathing. It consists of a combination of (1) obesity; (2) sleep-disordered breathing (SDB) in the form of obstructive sleep apnea hypopnea syndrome (OSAHS) with apnea–hypopnea index greater than 5 per hour and/or sleep hypoventilation syndrome (SHVS) (a 10–mm Hg increase in arterial PCO_2 or persistent oxygen desaturation not explained by obstructive apneas or hypopneas); and (3) stable daytime hypoventilation (arterial $PCO_2 > 45$ mm Hg).[72,73]

Most patients with OHS have OSAHS, but about 10% of patients have only SVHS.[74] OHS is associated with a higher morbidity and mortality rate compared with eucapnic OSAHS patients matched for age, body mass index, and lung function.[75] Patients with OHS make heavy use of health care resources with reduced use after treatment of OHS.[76]

Pathophysiology

Obesity is associated with reduced respiratory system compliance, increased airway resistance

attributed to a reduced functional residual capacity, and an increase in the work of breathing.[77,78] This increased load is associated with a perturbation of central respiratory drive in patients with OHS; they are unable to increase their respiratory drive in response to hypercapnia.[79] The causative role of SDB in OHS is seen by the improvement in wake hypercapnia after treatment of OSAHS and SHVS.[80–82] The precise mechanisms that predispose some patients with SDB to develop OHS are not clearly understood. Genetic factors have been proposed, but relatives of patients with OHS have not been reported to have abnormal ventilatory responses to hypercapnia.[83] A pivotal role for leptin in OSAHS has been suggested, because leptin-deficient mice have an impaired ventilatory response to hypercapnia before becoming obese.[84] In humans, the role of leptin in OHS has not been determined. Treatment of OSAHS in OHS patients has been shown to reduce OHS and leptin levels leading to speculation that OSAHS causes leptin resistance, and this leads to hypoventilation.[85] However, in OHS patients with SHVS and without OSAHS, treatment of SHVS has been reported to improve OHS and increase leptin levels, suggesting that SHVS may impair leptin production leading to daytime hypercapnia.[82]

How does SDB cause daytime hypoventilation? SDB results in intermittent hypercapnia with respiratory acidosis, resulting in renal metabolic compensation in the form of increased serum bicarbonate. This compensation has a long half-life that results in increased bicarbonate levels in the daytime. The persistent metabolic alkalosis is thought to blunt the central ventilatory response to carbon dioxide by reducing the change in hydrogen ions for a given change in carbon dioxide, in turn, leading to wake hypercapnia.[74]

Epidemiology

OHS is seen primarily in middle age with a male predominance that is not as prominent as in OSAHS, with an estimated prevalence of 10% to 20% of OSAHS patients that increases with degree of obesity.[74]

Clinical Features

Patients with OHS have symptoms suggestive of OSAHS such as fatigue, daytime somnolence, and loud snoring but are more likely to have dyspnea, daytime desaturation, and edema.[74] Serum bicarbonate is a useful screening test, and arterial blood gas testing usually reveals compensated respiratory acidosis with a normal pH.[73,74] Evaluation of lung functions is important to identify obstructive and restrictive lung disease. Patients with COPD and OSAHS (overlap syndrome) can have daytime hypercapnia. Conditions that can worsen hypoventilation, such as alcohol ingestion, also need to be identified.[73]

Management

Continuous positive airway pressure may be adequate to treat a subset of patients with OHS.[86] Patients who continue to have desaturation with CPAP should be provided BLPAP.[74] BLPAP in patients with OHS is provided as a form of noninvasive ventilation with the difference between inspiratory positive airway pressure and expiratory positive airway pressure being wide enough to provide adequate tidal volume.[80] Supplemental oxygen may be necessary if BLPAP does not correct oxygen desaturation. Monitoring compliance is an important component of management of patients with OHS because adherence to therapy of OHS is associated with improved outcomes.[74] Patients who do not tolerate noninvasive positive airway pressure should be considered for tracheostomy. Bariatric surgery, which can result in significant weight loss and improvement of OHS, may be appropriate for selected

patients but should be considered carefully because of attendant complications.[74]

OTHER ACQUIRED ALVEOLAR HYPOVENTILATION DISORDERS

Traumatic, ischemic, and inflammatory injuries in the brainstem region can result in acquired central hypoventilation. The term "Ondine's curse" was first used by Severinhaus and Mitchell[87] to describe patients who had minimal motor loss and retained the ability to breathe voluntarily after they underwent high bilateral spinothalamic tract cordotomies but became apneic during sleep and had poor ventilatory responsiveness to inhaled carbon dioxide. Unilateral lesions are less likely to have hypoventilation, and damage to C2 fibers is implicated in these cases.[88] Brainstem infarctions and ischemia can result in central hypoventilation syndromes.[89–91] Watershed infarcts in the brainstem tegmentum in the human fetal and neonatal brainstem can present with multiple cranial neuropathies, central hypoventilation and apnea, dysphagia and aspiration, Möbius syndrome, and Pierre Robin sequence.[91] Tumors in the region of the brain stem, such as glioma and acoustic neuroma, can lead to central hypoventilation.[92,93] Children with brain tumors often report sleepiness that may be related to central apneas or hypoventilation.[94] Hypoventilation may improve after tumor resection.[93] Bulbar polio and viral and paraneoplastic encephalitis have can occasionally result in central hypoventilation.[95–97] The outcome of acquired alveolar hypoventilation cases varies with the etiology and ventilatory management is usually supportive.

SUMMARY

Central alveolar hypoventilation disorders are rare and complex disorders that may involve alterations in mechanisms of ventilatory control and autonomic dysfunction. These disorders may be congenital or acquired and are associated with significant morbidity and mortality. For many years, the etiology of this group of disorders has not been well understood, and genetic characterization was a blank slate. Recently, CCHS has emerged as distinct neurodevelopmental disorder linked to mutations of the PHOX2B gene. It is anticipated that in the future genetic characterization will be available for other newly described disorders such as ROHHAD. Although respiratory abnormalities and autonomic dysfunction in patients with congenital central alveolar hypoventilation disorders persist throughout life, the prognosis for these children has improved considerably in recent years. This improvement may be attributed to wider recognition of such disorders, specialized centers treating such children, and improved technology to treat and monitor these children throughout life.

REFERENCES

1. Mellins RB, Balfour HH Jr, Turino GM, et al. Failure of automatic control of ventilation (Ondine's curse). Report of an infant born with this syndrome and review of the literature. Medicine (Baltimore) 1970; 49(6):487–504.
2. Nannapaneni R, Behari S, Todd NV, et al. Ondine's curse. Neurosurgery 2005;57(2):354–63 [discussion: 354–63].
3. Haddad GG, Mazza NM, Defendini R, et al. Congenital failure of automatic control of ventilation, gastrointestinal motility and heart rate. Medicine (Baltimore) 1978;57(6):517–26.
4. American Thoracic Society. Idiopathic congenital central hypoventilation syndrome: diagnosis and management. Am J Respir Crit Care Med 1999; 160(1):368–73.
5. Bower RJ, Adkins JC. Ondine's curse and neurocristopathy. Clin Pediatr (Phila) 1980;19(10):665–8.
6. Rohrer T, Trachsel D, Engelcke G, et al. Congenital central hypoventilation syndrome associated with Hirschsprung's disease and neuroblastoma: case of multiple neurocristopathies. Pediatr Pulmonol 2002;33(1):71–6.
7. Amiel J, Laudier B, Attie-Bitach T, et al. Polyalanine expansion and frameshift mutations of the paired-like homeobox gene PHOX2B in congenital central hypoventilation syndrome. Nat Genet 2003;33(4): 459–61.
8. Weese-Mayer DE, Berry-Kravis EM. Genetics of congenital central hypoventilation syndrome: lessons from a seemingly orphan disease. Am J Respir Crit Care Med 2004;170(1):16–21.
9. Vanderlaan M, Holbrook CR, Wang M, et al. Epidemiologic survey of 196 patients with congenital central hypoventilation syndrome. Pediatr Pulmonol 2004;37(3):217–29.
10. Trang H, Dehan M, Beaufils F, et al. The French congenital central hypoventilation syndrome registry: general data, phenotype, and genotype. Chest 2005;127(1):72–9.
11. Weese-Mayer DE, Silvestri JM, Menzies LJ, et al. Congenital central hypoventilation syndrome: diagnosis, management, and long-term outcome in thirty-two children. J Pediatr 1992;120(3):381–7.
12. Fleming PJ, Cade D, Bryan MH, et al. Congenital central hypoventilation and sleep state. Pediatrics 1980;66(3):425–8.
13. Child F, Couriel J. The control of breathing with reference to congenital central hypoventilation syndrome. J R Soc Med 1998;91(9):479–83.
14. Marcus CL, Bautista DB, Amihyia A, et al. Hypercapneic arousal responses in children with congenital central hypoventilation syndrome. Pediatrics 1991;88(5):993–8.
15. Paton JY, Swaminathan S, Sargent CW, et al. Hypoxic and hypercapnic ventilatory responses in awake children with congenital central hypoventilation syndrome. Am Rev Respir Dis 1989;140(2):368–72.
16. Shea SA, Andres LP, Shannon DC, et al. Respiratory sensations in subjects who lack a ventilatory response to CO2. Respir Physiol 1993;93(2):203–19.
17. Shea SA, Andres LP, Shannon DC, et al. Ventilatory responses to exercise in humans lacking ventilatory chemosensitivity. J Physiol 1993;468:623–40.
18. Silvestri JM, Weese-Mayer DE, Flanagan EA. Congenital central hypoventilation syndrome: cardiorespiratory responses to moderate exercise, simulating daily activity. Pediatr Pulmonol 1995; 20(2):89–93.
19. Paton JY, Swaminathan S, Sargent CW, et al. Ventilatory response to exercise in children with congenital central hypoventilation syndrome. Am Rev Respir Dis 1993;147(5):1185–91.
20. Shea SA, Andres LP, Paydarfar D, et al. Effect of mental activity on breathing in congenital central hypoventilation syndrome. Respir Physiol 1993; 94(3):251–63.
21. Gozal D, Marcus CL, Ward SL, et al. Ventilatory responses to passive leg motion in children with congenital central hypoventilation syndrome. Am J Respir Crit Care Med 1996;153(2):761–8.
22. Gozal D, Simakajornboon N. Passive motion of the extremities modifies alveolar ventilation during sleep in patients with congenital central hypoventilation syndrome. Am J Respir Crit Care Med 2000; 162(5):1747–51.
23. Chen ML, Keens TG. Congenital central hypoventilation syndrome: not just another rare disorder. Paediatr Respir Rev 2004;5(3):182–9.
24. Macey PM, Woo MA, Macey KE, et al. Hypoxia reveals posterior thalamic, cerebellar, midbrain, and limbic deficits in congenital central hypoventilation syndrome. J Appl Physiol 2005;98(3):958–69.
25. Harper RM, Macey PM, Woo MA, et al. Hypercapnic exposure in congenital central hypoventilation syndrome reveals CNS respiratory control mechanisms. J Neurophysiol 2005;93(3):1647–58.
26. Woo MS, Woo MA, Gozal D, et al. Heart rate variability in congenital central hypoventilation syndrome. Pediatr Res 1992;31(3):291–6.
27. Silvestri JM, Hanna BD, Volgman AS, et al. Cardiac rhythm disturbances among children with idiopathic congenital central hypoventilation syndrome. Pediatr Pulmonol 2000;29(5):351–8.

28. Trang H, Boureghda S, Denjoy I, et al. 24-hour BP in children with congenital central hypoventilation syndrome. Chest 2003;124(4):1393–9.

29. O'Brien LM, Holbrook CR, Vanderlaan M, et al. Autonomic function in children with congenital central hypoventilation syndrome and their families. Chest 2005;128(4):2478–84.

30. Cutz E, Ma TK, Perrin DG, et al. Peripheral chemoreceptors in congenital central hypoventilation syndrome. Am J Respir Crit Care Med 1997;155(1):358–63.

31. Trochet D, de Pontual L, Straus C, et al. PHOX2B Germline and Somatic Mutations in Late-Onset Central Hypoventilation Syndrome. Am J Respir Crit Care Med 2008;177(8):306–11.

32. Antic NA, Malow BA, Lange N, et al. PHOX2B mutation-confirmed congenital central hypoventilation syndrome: presentation in adulthood. Am J Respir Crit Care Med 2006;174(8):923–7.

33. Khalifa MM, Flavin MA, Wherrett BA. Congenital central hypoventilation syndrome in monozygotic twins. J Pediatr 1988;113(5):853–5.

34. Hamilton J, Bodurtha JN. Congenital central hypoventilation syndrome and Hirschsprung's disease in half sibs. J Med Genet 1989;26(4):272–4.

35. Silvestri JM, Chen ML, Weese-Mayer DE, et al. Idiopathic congenital central hypoventilation syndrome: the next generation. Am J Med Genet 2002;112(1):46–50.

36. Sritippayawan S, Hamutcu R, Kun SS, et al. Mother-daughter transmission of congenital central hypoventilation syndrome. Am J Respir Crit Care Med 2002;166(3):367–9.

37. Marazita ML, Maher BS, Cooper ME, et al. Genetic segregation analysis of autonomic nervous system dysfunction in families of probands with idiopathic congenital central hypoventilation syndrome. Am J Med Genet 2001;100(3):229–36.

38. Dubreuil V, Hirsch MR, Jouve C, et al. The role of Phox2b in synchronizing pan-neuronal and type-specific aspects of neurogenesis. Development 2002;129(22):5241–53.

39. Lo L, Morin X, Brunet JF, et al. Specification of neurotransmitter identity by Phox2 proteins in neural crest stem cells. Neuron 1999;22(4):693–705.

40. Pattyn A, Morin X, Cremer H, et al. The homeobox gene Phox2b is essential for the development of autonomic neural crest derivatives. Nature 1999;399(6734):366–70.

41. Sasaki A, Kanai M, Kijima K, et al. Molecular analysis of congenital central hypoventilation syndrome. Hum Genet 2003;114(1):22–6.

42. Weese-Mayer DE, Berry-Kravis EM, Zhou L, et al. Idiopathic congenital central hypoventilation syndrome: analysis of genes pertinent to early autonomic nervous system embryologic development and identification of mutations in PHOX2b. Am J Med Genet A 2003;123(3):267–78.

43. Stromme P, Mangelsdorf ME, Shaw MA, et al. Mutations in the human ortholog of aristaless cause X-linked mental retardation and epilepsy. Nat Genet 2002;30(4):441–5.

44. Berry-Kravis EM, Zhou L, Rand CM, et al. Congenital central hypoventilation syndrome: PHOX2B mutations and phenotype. Am J Respir Crit Care Med 2006;174(10):1139–44.

45. Matera I, Bachetti T, Puppo F, et al. PHOX2B mutations and polyalanine expansions correlate with the severity of the respiratory phenotype and associated symptoms in both congenital and late onset Central Hypoventilation syndrome. J Med Genet 2004;41(5):373–80.

46. Gronli JO, Santucci BA, Leurgans SE, et al. Congenital central hypoventilation syndrome: PHOX2B genotype determines risk for sudden death. Pediatr Pulmonol 2008;43(1):77–86.

47. Trochet D, O'Brien LM, Gozal D, et al. PHOX2B genotype allows for prediction of tumor risk in congenital central hypoventilation syndrome. Am J Hum Genet 2005;76(3):421–6.

48. Trang H, Laudier B, Trochet D, et al. PHOX2B gene mutation in a patient with late-onset central hypoventilation. Pediatr Pulmonol 2004;38(4):349–51.

49. Goldberg DS, Ludwig IH. Congenital central hypoventilation syndrome: ocular findings in 37 children. J Pediatr Ophthalmol Strabismus 1996;33(3):175–80.

50. Chen ML, Turkel SB, Jacobson JR, et al. Alcohol use in congenital central hypoventilation syndrome. Pediatr Pulmonol 2006;41(3):283–5.

51. Hays RM, Jordan RA, McLaughlin JF, et al. Central ventilatory dysfunction in myelodysplasia: an independent determinant of survival. Dev Med Child Neurol 1989;31(3):366–70.

52. Ward SL, Jacobs RA, Gates EP, et al. Abnormal ventilatory patterns during sleep in infants with myelomeningocele. J Pediatr 1986;109(4):631–4.

53. Kirk VG, Morielli A, Gozal D, et al. Treatment of sleep-disordered breathing in children with myelomeningocele. Pediatr Pulmonol 2000;30(6):445–52.

54. Swaminathan S, Paton JY, Ward SL, et al. Abnormal control of ventilation in adolescents with myelodysplasia. J Pediatr 1989;115(6):898–903.

55. Gozal D, Arens R, Omlin KJ, et al. Peripheral chemoreceptor function in children with myelomeningocele and Arnold-Chiari malformation type 2. Chest 1995;108(2):425–31.

56. Hertz G, Cataletto M, Feinsilver SH, et al. Sleep and breathing patterns in patients with Prader Willi syndrome (PWS): effects of age and gender. Sleep 1993;16(4):366–71.

57. Livingston FR, Arens R, Bailey SL, et al. Hypercapnic arousal responses in Prader-Willi syndrome. Chest 1995;108(6):1627–31.

58. Nixon GM, Brouillette RT. Sleep and breathing in Prader-Willi syndrome. Pediatr Pulmonol 2002; 34(3):209–17.

59. Arens R, Gozal D, Omlin KJ, et al. Hypoxic and hypercapnic ventilatory responses in Prader-Willi syndrome. J Appl Physiol 1994;77(5):2224–30.

60. Gozal D, Arens R, Omlin KJ, et al. Absent peripheral chemosensitivity in Prader-Willi syndrome. J Appl Physiol 1994;77(5):2231–6.

61. Arens R, Gozal D, Burrell BC, et al. Arousal and cardiorespiratory responses to hypoxia in Prader-Willi syndrome. Am J Respir Crit Care Med 1996; 153(1):283–7.

62. Van Vliet G, Deal CL, Crock PA, et al. Sudden death in growth hormone-treated children with Prader-Willi syndrome. J Pediatr 2004;144(1):129–31.

63. Sacco M, Di Giorgio G. Sudden death in Prader-Willi syndrome during growth hormone therapy. Horm Res 2005;63(1):29–32.

64. Nagai T, Obata K, Tonoki H, et al. Cause of sudden, unexpected death of Prader-Willi syndrome patients with or without growth hormone treatment. Am J Med Genet A 2005;136(1):45–8.

65. Bakker B, Maneatis T, Lippe B. Sudden death in Prader-Willi syndrome: brief review of five additional cases. [Concerning the article by U. Eiholzer et al.: deaths in children with Prader-Willi syndrome. A contribution to the debate about the safety of growth hormone treatment in children with PWS (Horm Res 2005;63:33–39)]. Horm Res 2007;67(4):203–4.

66. Craig ME, Cowell CT, Larsson P, et al. Growth hormone treatment and adverse events in Prader-Willi syndrome: data from KIGS (the Pfizer International Growth Database). Clin Endocrinol (Oxf) 2006; 65(2):178–85.

67. Festen DA, de Weerd AW, van den Bossche RA, et al. Sleep-related breathing disorders in prepubertal children with Prader-Willi syndrome and effects of growth hormone treatment. J Clin Endocrinol Metab 2006;91(12):4911–5.

68. Tauber M, Diene G, Molinas C, et al. Review of 64 cases of death in children with Prader-Willi syndrome (PWS). Am J Med Genet A 2008; 146(7):881–7.

69. Fishman LS, Samson JH, Sperling DR. Primary alveolar hypoventilation syndrome (Ondine's curse). Am J Dis Child 1965;110:155–61.

70. Katz ES, McGrath S, Marcus CL. Late-onset central hypoventilation with hypothalamic dysfunction: a distinct clinical syndrome. Pediatr Pulmonol 2000;29(1):62–8.

71. Ize-Ludlow D, Gray JA, Sperling MA, et al. Rapid-onset obesity with hypothalamic dysfunction, hypoventilation, and autonomic dysregulation presenting in childhood. Pediatrics 2007;120(1):e179–88.

72. Sleep-related breathing disorders in adults: recommendations for syndrome definition and measurement techniques in clinical research. The Report of an American Academy of Sleep Medicine Task Force. Sleep 1999;22(5):667–89.

73. Olson AL, Zwillich C. The obesity hypoventilation syndrome. Am J Med 2005;118(9):948–56.

74. Mokhlesi B, Tulaimat A. Recent advances in obesity hypoventilation syndrome. Chest 2007;132(4): 1322–36.

75. Hida W, Okabe S, Tatsumi K, et al. Nasal continuous positive airway pressure improves quality of life in obesity hypoventilation syndrome. Sleep Breath 2003;7(1):3–12.

76. Berg G, Delaive K, Manfreda J, et al. The use of health-care resources in obesity-hypoventilation syndrome. Chest 2001;120(2):377–83.

77. Rubinstein I, Zamel N, DuBarry L, et al. Airflow limitation in morbidly obese, nonsmoking men. Ann Intern Med 1990;112(11):828–32.

78. Sharp JT, Henry JP, Sweany SK, et al. The total work of breathing in normal and obese men. J Clin Invest 1964;43:728–39.

79. Han F, Chen E, Wei H, et al. Treatment effects on carbon dioxide retention in patients with obstructive sleep apnea-hypopnea syndrome. Chest 2001;119(6):1814–9.

80. de Lucas-Ramos P, de Miguel-Diez J, Santacruz-Siminiani A, et al. Benefits at 1 year of nocturnal intermittent positive pressure ventilation in patients with obesity-hypoventilation syndrome. Respir Med 2004;98(10):961–7.

81. Mokhlesi B, Tulaimat A, Evans AT, et al. Impact of adherence with positive airway pressure therapy on hypercapnia in obstructive sleep apnea. J Clin Sleep Med 2006;2(1):57–62.

82. Redolfi S, Corda L, La Piana G, et al. Long-term non-invasive ventilation increases chemosensitivity and leptin in obesity-hypoventilation syndrome. Respir Med 2007;101(6):1191–5.

83. Jokic R, Zintel T, Sridhar G, et al. Ventilatory responses to hypercapnia and hypoxia in relatives of patients with the obesity hypoventilation syndrome. Thorax 2000;55(11):940–5.

84. Tankersley C, Kleeberger S, Russ B, et al. Modified control of breathing in genetically obese (ob/ob) mice. J Appl Physiol 1996;81(2):716–23.

85. Yee BJ, Cheung J, Phipps P, et al. Treatment of obesity hypoventilation syndrome and serum leptin. Respiration 2006;73(2):209–12.

86. Banerjee D, Yee BJ, Piper AJ, et al. Obesity hypoventilation syndrome: hypoxemia during continuous positive airway pressure. Chest 2007;131(6):1678–84.

87. Severinghaus J, Mitchell R. Ondine's curse: failure of respiratory center automaticity while awake. Clin Res 1962;10:122.

88. Lahuerta J, Buxton P, Lipton S, et al. The location and function of respiratory fibres in the second cervical spinal cord segment: respiratory dysfunction syndrome after cervical cordotomy. J Neurol Neurosurg Psychiatry 1992;55(12):1142–5.

89. Bogousslavsky J, Khurana R, Deruaz JP, et al. Respiratory failure and unilateral caudal brainstem infarction. Ann Neurol 1990;28(5):668–73.

90. Smyth A, Riley M. Chronic respiratory failure: an unusual cause and treatment. Thorax 2002;57(9): 835–6.

91. Sarnat HB. Watershed infarcts in the fetal and neonatal brainstem. An aetiology of central hypoventilation, dysphagia, moibius syndrome and micrognathia. Eur J Paediatr Neurol 2004;8(2):71–87.

92. Lee DK, Wahl GW, Swinburne AJ, et al. Recurrent acoustic neuroma presenting as central alveolar hypoventilation. Chest 1994;105(3):949–50.

93. Hui SH, Wing YK, Poon W, et al. Alveolar hypoventilation syndrome in brainstem glioma with improvement after surgical resection. Chest 2000;118(1): 266–8.

94. Rosen GM, Bendel AE, Neglia JP, et al. Sleep in children with neoplasms of the central nervous system: case review of 14 children. Pediatrics 2003;112(1 Pt 1):e46–54.

95. Sarnoff SJ, Whittenberger JL, Affeldt JE. Hypoventilation syndrome in bulbar poliomyelitis. JAMA 1951;147(1):30–4.

96. White DP, Miller F, Erickson RW. Sleep apnea and nocturnal hypoventilation after western equine encephalitis. Am Rev Respir Dis 1983;127(1):132–3.

97. Vitaliani R, Mason W, Ances B, et al. Paraneoplastic encephalitis, psychiatric symptoms, and hypoventilation in ovarian teratoma. Ann Neurol 2005; 58(4):594–604.

98. Weese-Mayer DE, Silvestri JM, Huffman AD, et al. Case/control family study of autonomic nervous system dysfunction in idiopathic congenital central hypoventilation syndrome. Am J Med Genet 2001; 100(3):237–45.

99. Silvestri JM, Weese-Mayer DE, Nelson MN. Neuropsychologic abnormalities in children with congenital central hypoventilation syndrome. J Pediatr 1992;120(3):388–93.

100. Pine DS, Weese-Mayer DE, Silvestri JM, et al. Anxiety and congenital central hypoventilation syndrome. Am J Psychiatry 1994;151(6):864–70.

Index

Note: Page numbers of article titles are in **boldface** type.

A

Actigraph, measuring sleep in critically ill ICU
 patients, 572
Airway hyperreactivity, in relationship between
 asthma and obstructive sleep apnea, 508
Airway surgery, for obesity hypoventilation
 syndrome, 534
Alcohol, impairment of breathing during sleep due to,
 500
Amyotrophic lateral sclerosis, sleep disorders in, 544
Anesthetics, impairment of breathing during sleep
 due to, 500
Ankylosing spondylitis, extrapulmonary restriction in,
 518
Apnea. *See* Obstructive sleep apnea.
Architecture, sleep, effects of pharmacologic
 treatment in ICU patients on, 570–571
Arnold Chiari type II malformation, myelomeningocele
 with, hypoventilation in, 608
Arousal responses, impaired, in relationship between
 asthma and obstructive sleep apnea, 508
Asthma, bronchial, sleep and, in children, 589–590
 insomnia in, 581–583
  clinical epidemiology, 581
  clinical management of, 582–583
 disease impact on sleep, 582
 nocturnal, sleep physiology and, 501
 sleep and, 505–509
  epidemiology of sleep disorders in, 505–506
  pathogenesis of sleep disorders in, 506–507
   Circadian variations in lung function, 506
   gastroesophageal reflux, 507
   inflammatory changes at night, 506–507
   neurohormonal changes, 507
   variation in parasympathetic nervous
    system, 507
  relationship with obstructive sleep apnea,
   507–508
   corticosteroid therapy, 507–508
   gastroesophageal reflux disease, 508
   impaired arousal responses, 508
   increased airway hyperreactivity, 508
   inflammation, 508
   sinus disease, 508
   sleep fragmentation, 507
  sleep quality and, 508–509
Autonomic dysregulation, in rapid-onset obesity
 hypothalamic dysfunction and autonomic
 dysregulation, 609–610

B

Bariatric surgery, in obesity hypoventilation
 syndrome, 533–534
Behavioral management, if insomnia in respiratory
 diseases, 583–584
Bispectral index, measuring sleep in critically ill ICU
 patients, 572
Breathing, during sleep, medications and, 500–501
  drugs that can impair respiration, 500
  drugs that can stimulate respiration, 500–501
 effects of sleep on respiratory muscles and,
  541–542
Bronchial asthma, sleep and, in children, 589–590
Bronchopulmonary dysplasia. *See* Chronic lung
 disease of infancy.

C

Cardiovascular consequences, of sleep deprivation
 in critically ill ICU patients, 574
Central alveolar hypoventilation syndromes,
 congenital disorders, 601–609
  congenital central hypoventilation syndrome,
   601–608
  myelomeningocele with Arnold Chiari type II
   malformation, 608
  Prader-Willi syndrome, 608–609
 obesity hypoventilation syndrome, 610–611
 other acquired forms, 611
 rapid-onset obesity hypothalamic dysfunction and
  autonomic dysregulation, 609–610
Chest wall deformity, extrapulmonary restriction in,
 518
 insomnia in patients with, 583
Children, congenital central alveolar hypoventilation
 syndromes in, 601–609
  congenital central hypoventilation syndrome,
   601–608
  myelomeningocele with Arnold Chiari type II
   malformation, 608
  Prader-Willi syndrome, 608–609
 with respiratory disorders, sleep problems in,
  bronchial asthma, 589–590
  chronic lung disease of infancy,
   592–594
  cystic fibrosis, 590–592
  neuromuscular diseases, 596
  scoliosis, 595–596
  sickle-cell disease, 594–595

doi:10.1016/S1556-407X(08)00096-9

sleep.theclinics.com

Moving?

Make sure your subscription moves with you!

To notify us of your new address, find your **Clinics Account Number** (located on your mailing label above your name), and contact customer service at:

E-mail: elspcs@elsevier.com

800-654-2452 (subscribers in the U.S. & Canada)
314-453-7041 (subscribers outside of the U.S. & Canada)

Fax number: 314-523-5170

Elsevier Periodicals Customer Service
11830 Westline Industrial Drive
St. Louis, MO 63146

*To ensure uninterrupted delivery of your subscription, please notify us at least 4 weeks in advance of move.